The Fit Mom

Dawn Walters

ISBN: **1517682673**
ISBN-13: **978-1517682675**

DEDICATION

This book is dedicated to my mother, Trisha, who not only taught me, but showed me how to be an involved mother while also being a fit mom. She taught me how to eat healthy, make exercise a habit, and share both of those important lifestyle passions with her family. I couldn't have written this book without such an exquisite example as a part of my life. Thank you mom, for instilling in me a passion for parenting and fitness.

CONTENTS

INTRODUCTION

Let's face it- finding time to eat healthy and exercise amidst the hectic schedule of mothering can be difficult- to say the least. How do those fit moms do it? They must have some hidden secret they're not telling us about. Well, not exactly. Those 'fit moms' have just made a commitment to their health- and to their family's health for that matter. That's where being fit actually starts; by making a promise to yourself, and your family, that you want to eat well and be active.

Hold up, though- didn't I just say that eating healthy and exercising while parenting was really hard? Ya- I did. Trust me, I understand. That's why I'm writing "The Fit Mom" a simple, no-frills guide to creating a fit lifestyle for yourself and your family. No complicated diet plans. No crazy exercise regimens. No strict grocery lists, recipes, or work out equipment. Just 250 simple tips that everyone can follow.

THE FIT MOM

SETTING FITNESS GOALS

The first thing you need to do is decide what exactly you want to accomplish in terms of your fitness. Are you hoping to lose some weight, get in shape, get toned, or just feel better and have more energy? Whatever it is you want to accomplish- you need to set goals. Goals will keep you motivated and push you to better yourself each and every day. Every fitness guide will tell you- don't start out big. Start small. Walk a quarter of a mile, then a half mile, then a mile. Then run a mile. Then run two miles. Don't start out running two miles. Having small, manageable, achievable goals can work to your advantage in many ways.

In terms of exercising, working your way to where you want to go slowly allows your body to build up to the point you want it to go. If you haven't run a mile in the last year, and yet you decide randomly one day to run a mile- you're probably not going to be able to finish that mile in the condition you think you will. Your body needs to build up endurance. You need to let it get to a point, slowly, where it has the ability to run a mile.

Many people who dive head first into fitness also seem to get discouraged quickly. If you run a mile and wear out half-way through, because you haven't run a mile in a long time, you may give up. You'll say "I can't do it" and you'll quit. Set manageable fitness goals that you can achieve. With each goal you achieve you can push yourself a bit further. You'll keep yourself motivated, because you'll be constantly building yourself up to where you wish to be. The inspiration that comes from achieving small goals, will help you reach your big goal.

Your goals should not be focused on appearance. Appearance will follow performance. Your goals should be focused on what you're doing, rather than what you look like. If you hope to lose weight- that's great, but you shouldn't base your success on the number on the scale. Rather you should base success on what you've accomplished physically. Have you eaten healthy? Have you exercised regularly? Have you been working on reaching fitness goals? If all of these answer 'yes', then you are going to get fit. With that being said, appearance shouldn't be your focus. FEELING good should be your focus.

You should make a point to write down your goals for each day, week, and month. Daily- what do you hope to achieve? Do you want to eat a certain amount of vegetables? Do you want to run a certain distance or do a certain amount of exercises? Decide what your daily goals are. Each day, your goals should rise a bit. Start with 15 push-ups, then move onto 20. Build yourself up slowly. But each day you should have clear and concise goals that you hope to achieve.

Weekly you should also have goals. These goals should be more along the lines of breaking bad habits. Focus on one thing you hope to change that week. Maybe you'd like to replace 15 minutes of 'TV time' with a fitness activity.

Maybe you'd like to eat a healthier breakfast each day, or eliminate sugary drinks from your diet. Whatever it is, write down a goal each week to break one bad habit. Focusing on a single positive change for an entire week will give you a specific improvement to focus on. And one single improvement, at a time, is achievable. You can't change every bad habit at once, but you can certainly change every bad habit, one at a time. Take each week, and focus on one thing. One single thing you want to make better.

And lastly, you should have monthly goals. Monthly goals should basically reiterate your daily and weekly goals. This month did you; exercise 5 days a week? Eat healthy almost every single day? Achieve your weekly goals? Stick to your fitness plan? Each month you should track your progress. What did you do well on, and what can you improve on during the next month? Following your progress allows you to realize how much you've actually accomplished, and lets you figure out what you can improve on.

Speaking of accomplishing things- when you do accomplish a goal- reward yourself! By 'reward' I don't mean indulge in an unhealthy activity- like binge watching television or eating an entire cake. But do something you enjoy. Give yourself a hot bath, go buy yourself a shirt in a size smaller (that you can totally fit into now!), sip on a glass of wine while reading one of your favorite books (oh-oh, there's this great book called 'The Fit Mom' that would totally be perfect in this situation). Just do something you enjoy. Don't choose an unhealthy activity, and don't ruin the strides you've made with your 'reward'. But still take a moment to do something that makes you feel good. You're worth treating yourself to. And if you're constantly looking forward to your 'reward' for your hard work, you'll be motivated to work harder. Give yourself your own incentives to be better.

Having trouble sticking to your goals? Write them down! The visual effect of actually seeing and being reminded of your goals will help you stick to them. You'll be more likely to continue working on things if you can cross them off as you go. And each time you cross a 'task completed' off of your list, you'll have that little boost of seeing that you achieved a goal.

Keep your written goals in a place where you can see them. Hang them on the fridge, on your bathroom mirror, or taped to your work desk. Post them somewhere where you'll be forced to see them every day. You'll never have the excuse of you 'forgot' or it 'escaped your mind', because you had a physical reminder available to keep you on track.

Along with goals- you need to have a reason to accomplish those goals. A mere 'I'd like to look prettier' is probably not going to keep you motivated in the long term. Think bigger- better. There are SO many reasons to make a commitment to a healthy lifestyle. Being a healthier person in general opens up many more opportunities as a mother. You'll be healthier, and in so stand a better chance of living longer and being able to be a major part of your child's life well into adulthood. You'll also have more energy to do things with your kids. You'll stand as a positive health role model for your children- showing them how to live a productive lifestyle themselves when they grow up. And a healthy mom typically raises a very healthy family. If you're eating healthy and being active, your kids are going to be too. Fit people also tend to be more self-confident, and confidence is a great attribute to show your children you have. You'll show them that you can set goals and succeed in finishing them. Find reasons to be inspired, and focus on those reasons as a major part of your new fitness lifestyle.

EATING

Being healthy on the outside, starts with being healthy on the inside. That old saying, "You are what you eat" holds true in modern times more than ever. We have greasy, sugary, salty foods available at our disposal. We have more unhealthy foods available than we have healthy foods. Unhealthy foods are more accessible, more convenient, and often we crave them because they taste good. In order to eat healthy, we have to consciously make the decision to do so- and put in the effort to make healthy eating a priority for ourselves and our family.

You won't eat healthy if those around you also are not eating healthy. It's important that you make healthy eating a family activity. If everyone else in your household is eating TV dinners, you're not going to feel satisfied munching on your salad. The best way to avoid temptation is to not be around temptation. And let's face it- feeding your family healthier isn't a bad idea.

Planning Meals

There is a common misconception that eating healthy involves a time commitment. That's not necessarily true. There are many convenient, easy ways to eat healthy. But they do require an effort and some additional planning. Speaking of planning, a family that eats healthy typically has a meal plan. They plan out their meals a week or a month in advance. Creating a meal plan will give you the tools you need to eat healthy at every single meal, every single day.

Weekly meal plans work best. Each day you should have planned out your breakfast, lunch, and dinner. You should also plan out additional healthy snack items that you and your family can eat in-between meals. When planning meals opt for well-balanced meals. Meals that include a good amount of protein (meat) and vegetables- as well as some whole grains, fruits, and dairy. Protein will keep you fuller longer, and give you energy throughout the day. Grains on the other hand tend to give you a lot of energy right away, but don't provide long-term fulfillment or energy. Opting for meals comprised mostly of meat, rather than grains will keep your family fuller, longer. Focusing on sides of fruits and vegetables will help your family get necessary nutrients and vitamins. Dairy and grains are also necessary, but because of their high fat and carb contents, shouldn't be the main focus of the meals.

Fresh foods are best. When possible avoid frozen, canned, processed, and dried foods. Most of these pre-packaged foods tend to include additional preservatives and flavor-additives that aren't necessarily healthy. If you'd like to cook with freezer meals, opt for making your own meals at home, freezing them, and cooking them later on. That way you know exactly what went into the meal you're cooking and no unnecessary unhealthy items were added. We'll discuss more about freezer meals, and how they can benefit your healthy eating regimen later in this chapter.

Avoid unhealthy quick meals. Any meal that needs to be prepared out of a package, box, or can- probably isn't the best option. A lot of people believe that these meals are budget friendly. And, to be honest, they love the convenience of a two minute preparation time. They may take a few minutes less to prepare, but the misconception that they are more affordable just isn't true. You can absolutely shop healthy within your budget. But you need to change the way you look at finances and food.

Why Your Budget Is Hurting Your Diet Success

Yes- your obsession with your bank account can definitely be hurting your chances at eating healthy. You probably didn't realize it. You've been crunching numbers and obsessing over grocery prices. So you didn't take the time to think that possibly, the reason you're not eating as healthy as you should- is that you're not making the financial investment you need to in order to eat healthy. Eating healthy doesn't cost more money. That's a myth- and it's been busted. BUT you think it costs more money, because there are a lot of things you don't factor in when budgeting our grocery list. Well, it's time to start becoming aware of your finances AND your food habits. Here are a few misconceptions you probably don't even realize you have. But the next time you're writing your grocery list, keep these in mind.

Fast Food Is Not Cheaper Food

That $4.00 box of fried chicken may look like a good deal compared to the package of fresh unseasoned drumsticks at the same price, but chances are you're getting way less meat and way more cheap fillers in that package of fried chicken. All of that breading and seasoning is there for a reason- and once you pull it away you're left with 1/3 of the meat you thought was there. Don't be fooled by the bigger box- you're most likely getting the same amount of meat in that package of fresh chicken wings as you are in the fried ones. The only difference is that one is coated in greasy unhealthy breading and the other is

Processed Foods Don't Save Money

Chips are on sale! We gotta buy some. Oh- and Oreos too! While we're at it, let's just walk down the entire over-processed food aisle and fill our cart with every dang thing that's cheap. We can eat it all! Mwah ha ha ha haaa. Stop-stop it right there. Yes, chips are cheap. But chips don't fill you up. You'll eat that entire bag of chips and STILL be hungry. On the other hand, a little pricier but more fulfilling option would be a set of bananas. They're filled with vitamins and nutrients that will leave you feeling fuller significantly longer than chips would. So, really, you're getting your money's worth with the bananas, while you're simply temporarily fixing your appetite with chips. Which one is -actually- the smarter investment?

Organics Aren't Out Of Your Price Range

We have this misconception that organics are expensive. Ya, they're a bit pricier- but you don't need to buy everything organic. Buy the foods you use the most in organic form. If your family drinks a lot of milk- try budgeting organic milk into your groceries. Same goes for different veggies and meat. You don't need to go 100% organic to eat organic. Pick the foods that mean the most to you, and budget them in. You'll feel good about it, and the food you're eating will be a little bit healthier.

You Look For Deals Rather Than Meals

If you're an avid coupon user, chances are you're obsessed with finding a good deal rather than a complete meal. So fresh lettuce is on sale! You buy three heads of lettuce. But unless you eat lettuce regularly you're probably wasting your money. That lettuce will go bad and you'll have wasted your money on one cheap sale item instead of spreading it out over an array of healthier items. Instead of buying in bulk just because something is on sale- stick to a meal plan. Create balanced meals, list out their ingredients- and then search for coupons for those specific ingredients. You're then getting deals on foods you'll actually eat, rather than things that are simply cheap but you won't necessarily use.

You See Ingredients Prices Rather Than Portion Prices

When you look at the price of individual products you see the total price of an ingredient rather than a meal. So let's say you buy the meat, sauce, cheese, and noodles needed for lasagna. All of those ingredients separately can add up to a hefty total. Or you could buy a cheaper microwave meal for 1/5 the cost. What you don't realize is that the microwave meal is one serving. All of the ingredients for the lasagna make up many servings. Per serving the lasagna is much less expensive. Quit focusing on the price of individual products and start focusing on portion price-you'll see that homemade is cheaper than microwaved 100% of the time.

So, yes, maybe your financial awareness is ruining your attempts at eating healthy. But it doesn't have to. Taking a few of these ideas into account when creating your grocery budget can make a world of change. Eating healthy is an investment, but it doesn't have to break the bank. You can be money-smart and food-smart at the same time, as long as you don't let one mentality overrun the other.

Once you realize that your budget and healthy eating can go hand in hand, you open up a lot of healthy eating opportunities for yourself. Say goodbye to boxed meals and prepackaged foods and hello to fresh, organic, wholesome ingredients that are well-worth making a meal out of.

Another argument many people will make is that "My family doesn't like healthy foods". If you have a picky eater raise your hand. Me too! Trust me- a lot of parents out there have picky eaters. Ya, we can feed our picky eaters Doritos all day long to conveniently satisfy their hunger without forcing green beans down their throat. OR we can make the green beans just as appealing than the Doritos. Compared to the cheesy crunchy goodness of Doritos, even the most health-conscious adults aren't going to enjoy nibbling on a green bean instead. Unless you make that green bean just as appealing. Get creative in your cooking. Don't settle for bland flavors. Ever fried green beans in taco seasoning? Sooo good! And –bam- green beans all of the sudden aren't that bad. In fact, they're pretty yummy. You need to be willing to look at bland healthy foods and figure out how to make them taste better. For your family's sake, and for yours. Healthy foods CAN be appealing.

Additionally- there are probably a ton of healthy foods your family already likes. Almost all kids love fruit. And if you gave them a bowl of blueberries rather than a package of fruit snacks, they'd be equally as happy. The crunch of celery with the sweetness of peanut butter on top is a great convenient snack that beats potato chips any day. Trust me, when you start walking down the 'fresh produce' aisle, rather than rummaging in the snack aisle, you'll realize there are a lot of very delicious foods you've been purposely skipping over. It's time to start picking up the healthy options instead. Your taste buds won't miss candy bars once they are spoiled by eating fruit every day.

Go to the grocery store and pick out healthy foods that you like. If you love salmon- buy salmon. If you love watermelon buy watermelon. The point is, that once you begin looking at healthy foods you'll realize there are a lot of healthy foods you crave and actually enjoy eating. Many people think they don't want to eat healthy. They think they're craving Chef Boyardee and Banquet Chicken. In reality, once they go to the aisle where there's yummy fish fillets and salad mixes and decadent fruits instead- they'll realize that they definitely want to eat those things. Healthy food isn't always gross or bland. It's just something that we forget we want, because we're looking down the aisle of cereal boxes instead.

Speaking of liking healthy foods- buy what you like. If you choose to buy healthy foods, just because they're healthy, you're going to be miserable eating them. If you hate broccoli, don't buy broccoli. Buy foods you actually like and want to eat. It will make eating healthy so much easier when you actually like the healthy options you're buying for yourself. You can also find healthy alternatives to practically any meal. If you love lasagna- learn how to make lasagna from scratch with whole grain noodles, home-made pasta sauce, and fresh cheeses. It will taste better, it won't be ridden with preservatives and additives, and it will be so much healthier for you. Another plus side to making your own lasagna from scratch? You can do so ahead of time, and freeze it. In fact you can freeze SO many meals and cook them throughout the week. Taking a few hours on Sunday to pre-make a few meals, will help you have quick and easy options when you get busier later in the week.

There are a lot of healthy meals that are easy to prepare. Baked salmon, grilled chicken breasts, mashed potatoes, steamed veggies, and mixed fruits are just a few options. If there are a few specific healthy meals that you enjoy, and can prepare quickly and efficiently- make them your 'family staples'. Choose a few meals each week that you can prep easily. Eating healthy shouldn't require extravagant recipes and hard work. Choose foods that are convenient for you. Find meals you like, that are easy to prepare, and that you WANT to make and eat. When you're making healthy foods that require minimum work, but have maximum taste appeal- you're going to eat healthier more often.

Choose healthy snack options. As you're shopping not only should you be thinking about creating three balanced meals a day, but also purchasing items that you and your family can snack on between meals. Everyone snacks- everyone naturally gets hungry at random times throughout the day. Don't resort to potato chips and candy bars at that time. Instead focusing on finding items that would be better suited for your new healthy lifestyle. Protein bars, dried fruits, nuts, veggie chips, and popcorn are just a few quick and semi-healthy options.

Shop Smart

Shopping with the intent of eating healthy is vitally important. Your 'shopping time' determines whether or not you actually eat healthy the rest of the week. If you go into the store and pick up chips, candy, cereal, and microwave meals ALONG with your healthy foods, you're going to eat the unhealthy foods. They're convenient, and they're available. Avoid the unhealthy foods at all cost. Don't even put them in your cart. Don't look at them. Write a list of all of the ingredients you need for each meal of the week, as well as a collection of healthy snack items. And STICK TO THAT LIST! Do not waver. Do not spontaneously add other things to your cart (unless they're healthy). Seriously- avoid the unhealthy foods. I know it's hard. Every time I enter a grocery store I struggle with the battle to march right down the cereal aisle and buy a box of Fruit Loops. What do they put in Fruit Loops? Some magical sweetener that makes them so dang good? But I don't- I don't buy the Fruit Loops. I stick to my list, and by the time I get home, my kitchen is filled with only healthy, delicious options that my family and I can enjoy all week long.

There's an old saying that you should never go grocery shopping on an empty stomach, and it has a legitimate reasoning behind it. When your stomach is empty it begins to crave foods- usually high fat, high sugar, unhealthy foods. When your stomach is craving food, even the most strong-willed of individuals can fall into the 'spontaneously buying an unhealthy item' trap. Eating before you go grocery shopping, will prevent your stomach from controlling your mind. Instead you'll be able to stick to a rational thought process and only buy what's on your list.

The edges of the grocery store are typically where all of the healthy items are offered. Fresh fruits, vegetables, meats, fish, and dairy products are all stored around the edges. On the other hand over-processed, boxed, and prepackaged foods are stored in the middle. You can completely avoid those 'over-processed foods', by instead focusing a large majority of your shopping trip on the edges of the store. Always start your grocery shopping list by walking around the very outer edges of the store, filling your cart with everything that's offered on the list. Then, you can find any remaining items in the inner aisles. Don't merely walk through every single inner aisle though. Find the one that has the item you're looking for and go straight to that item. This will help you avoid 'strolling and picking'- essentially just walking through the aisle and spontaneously finding an item you'd like to purchase and adding it to your cart- even though it may not be healthy or on your grocery list.

I love grocery shopping with my children. It's a great activity for them, and we have a lot of fun picking out fruits and vegetables and things as a family. With that being said, my kids certainly do tend to beg- for everything. They'll see a bag of Cheetos and beg for Cheetos. Lucky Charms? They'll beg for those too. Kraft Mac n' Cheese- yep, it's a favorite in our household. With kids constantly pointing out tempting unhealthy food items, I often find myself buying something unhealthy merely to shut them up- or because they pointed out something that appealed to me. If your kids do tend to beg while grocery shopping, it may be best to leave them at home- especially if you're not feeling strong-willed enough that day to say "No" at every salty, greasy, sugary item you pass.

With that being said, when you do take your children grocery shopping- stick to the edges of the store and get them excited about picking out different healthy items. Let them choose which bunch of bananas to buy, or teach them how to judge the ripeness of an avocado. Instill in them healthy food choices and let them be a part of the shopping process. When your children become MORE excited about buying produce than breakfast cereal- you've just inspired a very healthy eating mindset in them.

There are a few places where it's absolutely appropriate to get a bit 'spontaneous' in your shopping. Healthy snack items like fruits, vegetables, salad mixes, nuts, dried fruits, and dried vegetables are almost all worthwhile investments. If you see a fruit in season that you don't have on your list- but you're craving, pick it up. It's a FRUIT! It's good for you! Same goes for spontaneously trying any new healthy food or picking up a bag of your favorite nuts. As long as the item isn't over-processed and is obviously healthy, 'spontaneous shopping' isn't a bad thing. Just don't spontaneously buy things that are obviously not good for you.

Writing a list and sticking to it helps you in a variety of ways, but one of the biggest ways it can benefit you is by limiting your trips to the grocery store. When you buy an entire week's worth of ingredients for meals, you prevent additional trips to the grocery store. Every time you enter a grocery store there are aisles and aisles (and check out displays) of temptations. Unhealthy temptations. On the other hand, at home- in your kitchen where you control what is available, there doesn't have to be temptation. By purchasing enough items each week to fulfill all of your snack and mealtime needs, you're ensuring that for an entire week you're eating healthy. You've made a commitment to yourself by buying all of the healthy items and fully stocking your kitchen with them.

EATING HEALTHY WITH YOUR FAMILY

So, now your kitchen is stocked and full of healthy food items. You've gotten in the habit of creating meal plans, writing grocery lists, and purchasing and cooking healthy foods. BUT, the hardest part of having a healthy lifestyle, is matching it to your family's preferences. As your child ages, they will develop different eating habits. Eating healthy as a family changes as the family grows and develops.

There are many different stages your child will go through, and your 'healthy eating' habits will change as you go through those stages with them. So let's start at the beginning. Pregnancy.

While Pregnant

Pregnancy is by far one of the hardest times to maintain a healthy eating regimen, and yet it's one of the most important times to do so. Your body needs as many nutrients, vitamins, and minerals that you can provide it during that time. It's important to understand that your body will need additional food during this time, and it's natural to crave very high-fat items. Dairy items are great for curing this craving, and upping your dairy content during pregnancy can be very beneficial to your health. Unlike most fatty foods- like, potato chips, French fries, and shakes- dairy products are not unhealthy for you. They'll cure your craving for high-fat items without diminishing your health. Not only does dairy have a high fat content, it's also very high in calcium- which is good for both you and the baby blossoming within your belly. Iodine is another very important vitamin during pregnancy in terms of helping your child's brain and nervous system develop appropriately, and many dairy products like milk and cottage cheese have significant amounts of iodine in them. Typically, when you are not pregnant you will want to limit your dairy intake because of its high fat content, but while pregnant it is very good for you to focus a large portion of your diet on dairy items for their calcium and iodine contents.

Fruits and vegetables should always be a main staple of your diet, but even more so while you are pregnant. Different produce are packed with different vitamins and minerals, so eating a variety each day is very good for you. Upping your vitamin C intake by focusing on foods like oranges, grapefruits, strawberries, papaya, tomatoes, broccoli, and green peppers will help you stay healthy and help your baby grow strong. Leafy vegetables like spinach and loose-leaf lettuce mixes have folic acid- another beneficial vitamin. Many vegetables like carrots, sweet potatoes, and pumpkins have vitamin A in them- which is another great vitamin to aid your baby in their growth.

Upping your fiber and iron intakes during pregnancy are also very healthy for you. Breakfast cereals, oatmeal, and beans all have both high contents of fiber and iron. Specifically for women who struggle with constipation during pregnancy, adding additional fiber-rich foods to your diet can help you regulate your digestive system.

Eating a variety of foods is what is key here. Just as when you're not pregnant, focusing on healthy, natural, fresh, organic options are best. You want to focus on eating well, eating well-balanced, and eating a variety. While pregnant there is no better time to raid the fresh food aisle. Pick up an array of fruits and veggies and munch on them as often as you'd like. They'll benefit both you and your baby.

Morning Sickness

For the many women out there who struggle with morning sickness- eating a well-balanced diet can seem nearly impossible. Eating anything can feel impossible. There is no worse feeling than feeling sick... all the time. If you tend to struggle with morning sickness try munching on some whole wheat crackers or whole wheat toast first thing in the morning. It will give your stomach a light meal that shouldn't overwhelm your digestive system, but should help you get the energy you need to begin the day.

Throughout the day focus on eating multiple small meals rather than three basic meals. Split your meals up into much smaller portions and focus on 'light' foods such as chicken, turkey, leafy vegetables, melons, citrus fruits, berries, eggs, applesauce, bread, oatmeal, and mild cheeses. Avoid heavier items when you're feeling sick. Things like greasy meats (steak and ground beef), potatoes, noodles, over-processed foods, and milk can sometimes make your stomach feel even worse.

Cravings

To the contrast of morning sickness and simply not wanting to eat- comes food cravings. Statistics have shown that nearly 2/3 of all pregnant women will experience some kind of food craving. Typically this is your body telling you that it needs a specific nutrient, and it knows it can receive that nutrient from the food you are craving. If you have the urge to eat a specific food (mozzarella cheese, pickles, watermelon, raisons, or eggs are a few common examples) eat that food. Indulge yourself. With that being said, you should also be eating other foods to create a well-balanced diet for yourself. Eat a variety of foods, but when you get a craving it's absolutely reasonable to eat the food that you have the urge to eat.

You should be attuned to your body's cravings, but if you are craving something unhealthy (deep fried chicken, Oreo cookies, etc) then try to find alternative foods to replace the item you're craving. Here are a few healthy alternatives for different cravings…

Salty: Pickles, nuts, sunflower seeds, hard cheeses,

Sweet: Peanut butter on wheat toast, dried fruits, fresh fruits, smoothies, yogurt

Chocolate: Chocolate milk, dried fruit, one square of dark chocolate, cherries, dried coconut

Fatty: Cottage cheese, milk, ground beef, popcorn, pumpkin seeds

No-No Foods

During pregnancy there are some foods that should be avoided. Alcohol is obviously something you need to completely eliminate from your pregnancy diet. Studies have shown the many dangers of ingesting alcohol while pregnant and by doing so you are putting your baby at a major risk.

Aside from alcohol, your caffeine intake should also be limited. Yes, this means kicking your beloved coffee, tea, soda, and chocolate to the curb for a while. All four of these things are high in caffeine, which is not beneficial to you or your child during pregnancy.

Any fish that are high in mercury should also be avoided. You should not eat tilefish, mackerel, shark, or swordfish while pregnant, as the mercury content within them has been proven to cause significant problems for growing fetuses. Raw fish also pose the risk of food-borne illness and shellfish poisoning. Any raw fish should not be eaten, but shellfish (like raw oysters) should especially be avoided.

Lastly, soft cheeses like feta and brie should be avoided when possible, unless they are advertised as being pasteurized. Typically these cheeses are unpasteurized and risk the chance of causing a Listeria infection. Appropriate replacements for soft cheese cravings would be cottage cheese, cream cheese, parmesan, and mozzarella cheeses.

Eating Healthy All Nine Months

Having the goal to eat healthy during all nine months of your pregnancy will make pregnancy a healthier experience and give your child a healthier start to life. Continue to write down meal plans and stick to shopping lists when you are pregnant. The positive habits you created prior to pregnancy shouldn't end just because you're growing a kiddo in your belly. Continue to make an effort to eat healthy, on purpose, as often as possible.

Shop healthy

Even amidst morning sickness and food cravings, your ultimate goal when you go into the grocery store should be to walk out with a cart full of healthy items that will allow you to eat a well-balanced diet. Continue to skip over the convenient pre-packaged foods. Your body will thank you for it later.

Have your family eating healthy as well

It's extremely difficult to eat healthy when those around you are not eating healthy. Request that your spouse also make an effort to eat a well-balanced diet with you. Preparing well-balanced diets for both of you, and eating a healthy diet together will benefit you both. If you have other children in the home, keeping them on the same well-balanced diet you're eating will help you manage meal plans easier and provide healthy options for both you and your little ones.

Keep an array of healthy foods on stock

Pregnancy cravings strike at the weirdest times. And the urge to eat- a lot, happens quite often. Rather than running out to the grocery store at midnight (or even worse- the nearest fast food restaurant) keep a healthy array of snacks constantly available. For long-term storage dried berries, sunflower seeds, pumpkin seeds, coconut flakes, dried fruits, nuts, cheeses, peanut butter, and whole wheat crackers are great things to keep on stock. You never know when you'll have the urge to munch, and having healthy things to munch on available will keep you on your right healthy-eating track.

With Your Baby

Breastfeeding

Eating well with a baby may be the easiest time in your life to eat healthily. If you can breastfeed, do breastfeed. There are so many benefits to breastfeeding. It's obviously very nutritional for your child and helps your baby grow with the natural vitamins that they need. It's also a magnificent bonding activity, reducing stress for both you and your child. Along with the mental and physical benefits-breastfeeding is a calorie burning machine. There is no more convenient way to burn off baby fat than to breastfeed your baby. Your body will be burning calories practically faster than you can draw them in.

With that being said, burning fat and losing weight should not be your primary concern (or even your goal) while breastfeeding. Rather, you're main goal should be to continue to eat healthy, eat well, and supply your baby with the nutrients they need to grow big and strong. As always, a well-balanced diet is important. A good array of fruits, vegetables, meats, dairy products, and whole grains will give you the energy to care for your little one- and give you the vitamins you need to produce the best possible milk for them.

An array of flavors in the food you eat- including spicy foods can help introduce your child to new flavors through your breast milk and make your child more acceptable to new foods once they've moved onto solids. Eat an array of foods and keep your breast milk full of an array of vitamins, nutrients, and flavors that will help your baby grow physically, and mentally.

Unlike during pregnancy when dairy products were very beneficial for you- those same saturated fats aren't going to benefit you nearly as much while breast feeding. Yes, you still need a good amount of calcium, but you won't necessarily need to eat a larger amount of dairy because of this. With that being said 'good fats' like fats from canola oil, olive oil, avocados, nuts, and seeds are great for you during this time. These will help provide your baby with the fatty-nutrients they need without causing you to put on extra pounds.

Omega 3s from fish are also very important for your child's development and upping your intake of certain fish while breastfeeding can give you a good amount of energy from the protein, while also supplying your child with omega-3 fats that can help in nervous system development. Some fish, like we discussed in the pregnancy section, are high in mercury and because of this should be avoided. Swordfish, mackerel, shark, and tilefish are the most dangerous. Albacore tuna and solid white tuna also tend to have higher mercury percentages. Opt for light tuna instead. Omega-3 rich fish that are healthy for you while breastfeeding include many sea foods such as scallops, crab, shrimp, tilapia, salmon, and Pollack. Many freshwater fish such as lake trout and catfish are also good.

Just as while pregnant, alcohol should be avoided when possible. Although many medical experts will say that in moderation alcohol will not hurt during breastfeeding- remember that everything you put into your body (including the toxins of alcohol) while breastfeeding, stand a chance of being passed onto your child. For the same reason items high in caffeine (such as coffee, tea, soda, chocolate, and energy drinks) should also be avoided or limited to a minimum amount- and only indulged in occasionally, not regularly.

Most women are going to feel a bit hungrier than usual while breastfeeding. Unlike while carrying a baby, you do not need to be putting on additional weight (or eating significantly more calories) while breastfeeding. Eat three well balanced meals a day. To avoid overeating, eat light snacks between meals. It will prevent the hunger from causing you to binge-eat, while also preventing you from eating too many calories throughout the day.

Solid Foods

As your baby transitions from breast milk (or formula) to solid foods, you can work on creating a healthy diet for them, and letting their diet inspire your own eating habits. As often as possible you should focus on making your own homemade baby food. A food puree'er will quickly become your best friend. Use organic wholesome ingredients and create a variety of foods for your baby to try. Having a diverse array of foods for your child's pallet will help them become more accustomed to new flavors- and more keen on trying new foods later in life. Making your child healthy baby food from scratch will also help you eat better. Typically you'll be eating what your child is eating. Chicken with a light gravy, sweet potatoes, applesauce, peas, pears, beef stew. There are an array of foods that you can puree for your child and also eat yourself. You'll notice, as you make baby food, that you limit the ingredients you add. You focus on one to three sole ingredients for the entire meal. You don't add extra salt, preservatives, additives, and unhealthy substitutes. You do this to create a healthier meal for your child, but if you share those meals with your child- you will also be creating a healthier meal for yourself.

Sharing healthy wholesome meals with your baby as they transition to solid foods is a great way to help begin to get rid of any additional baby fat your body may still have stored. Your meals should be based on meats, fruits, vegetables, light grains, and light dairy products. The large amount of meats and fruits and vegetables will keep your body happy and healthy, but the minimal grains and dairy products will avoid unnecessary carbs and fats- which will help you lose any of that additional baby weight as soon as possible.

Try to eat what your baby eats as often as possible, and focus on healthy foods made with organic ingredients. Every mother wants their child to grow big and strong- and a well-balanced fresh food diet can help accomplish that. At the same time though, many mothers choose not to feed themselves those same well-balanced fresh food diets, which they need to stay healthy and strong. Be the mom that shares her healthy meal plan with her child, rather than simply creating a healthy meal plan for her child and not herself.

With Your Kids

As your child grows up, creating healthy food habits from a young age is very important. The best way to accomplish a healthy attitude towards food in your children? Have a healthy attitude towards food yourself. Children follow their parent's behavior. Set a good example for your child by eating healthy in front of them, making homemade meals with natural ingredients, and focusing on the importance of what you put within your body.

Why You, As A Parent, Should Eat What You Feed Your Kids

Let's face it, we love our kids- and because we love them, we try to feed them well. We want them to be healthy happy young individuals, so we give them every opportunity to succeed by making sure their nutritional needs are covered and their bodies are well taken care of. The real question is- why aren't we doing the same things for ourselves? We should be treating or bodies the same way we treat our kid's. What we have on our plate should be the same exact thing our kids have on theirs.

You Feed Them A Well-Balanced Diet
Chances are you know exactly the nutrition's your kid needs. Meat, grains, vegetables, fruits, and dairy are all a part of their diet. They should be a part of your diet too. We want our children to be fed an array of foods that are good for them, but we often don't do the same thing for ourselves. Watch what you eat, and make sure you also get an array of healthy foods in your diet.

You Watch Their Sugar Intake
Everyone knows the old myth (or should I say truth?) that kids get hyper when fed sugar. So we watch their candy intake carefully. Ice cream is a special treat, not a daily snack. And if they do get candy bars or something full of hyper-ness causing sweetness, we budget their intake. They definitely don't get to eat as much as they want. And we

shouldn't either. We need to start budgeting our own sugar intake. Too much of anything isn't good for you. And we all know too much sugar isn't good for us.

You Watch Their Caffeine Intake Too

Along with sugar, one thing we know we can't feed our kids in bulk is caffeine. Yet we as adults seem to develop an addiction to this amazing energy-giving clutch. But just as we treat our children, we should treat ourselves and we should monitor how much coffee, pop, and tea we put in our systems. Just as with sugar- too much caffeine can cause a lot of issues for us, and we should be portioning ourselves the same way we portion our kids.

You Make Sure They Eat Their Veggies

Yes, even if they hate the bland taste you sit there and make sure they eat every little last bite of those good-for-them vegetables. Why don't you do the same thing for yourself? You deserve those nutrient-packed vitamin-holding plants in your system as well. They promote good health in so many ways, so every time you tell your kids to eat their vegetables you should start telling yourself to do the same.

You Make Them Take Their Vitamins

As you grow older you don't grow out of a need for vitamins, and many adults forget that (until we reach 50 and our doctors begin reminding us again). Needless to say a vitamin a day is never a bad approach to take to your health. And if you're inspired by your kids chewables, there are the same gummy-style versions for adults. You have no excuse not to take a vitamin each day.

We need to begin to treat our bodies the same way we would treat our child's. We want our kids to grow and be strong, but we should want ourselves to stay strong.

Strength comes from within, and what you put in your body means a lot in terms of your health (both mental and physical). So start taking a lesson from your mom and dad, and make yourself eat the way your parents would want you to.

Every family has different taste preferences. Every child has different taste preferences. Just as you don't like every single food, nor does your child. Focus on creating healthy meals that everyone likes. Healthy eating shouldn't mean that everyone in the family has to eat foods they don't enjoy. It should mean that you work together to create healthy meals that everyone wants to sit down to feast upon. If your family loves sweet potatoes, then make sweet potatoes often. If your family is a huge fan of salmon- make salmon often. Healthy eating doesn't need to be complicated. Make a point to cook what you and your family want to eat.

Make healthy foods a habit. Healthy eating shouldn't be a 'few times a week' event. Healthy eating should just be a basic part of your family's lifestyle. You eat healthy every single meal, every single day. It's not merely a 'phase', it's a lifestyle. Once you get in the habit of eating healthy, regularly, as a family- eating healthy is no longer a chore, but an enjoyable activity that makes you feel good inside and out. Don't simply try to eat healthy 'every once in a while'. Eat healthy ALL the time.

A common misconception many people have is that in order to eat healthy they need to give up foods that they love. And that's just not true. There are healthy alternatives to literally every single food out there. Love French fries? Try homemade baked fries rather than frozen deep-fried fries. They taste just as good, but are so much healthier for you. Don't assume that the foods you love don't have healthy alternatives. Everything from chocolate cake to pizza to chicken nuggets has a way to be made healthily. It just takes a bit of research, and a willingness to change had habits.

Have set meal times with your family. Eating three basic meals at regular times each day will help your family get on a healthy-eating regimen. It will help you avoid overeating and indulging in unhealthy snacks. It will also help you accurately plan out different meals throughout the day. Having set times to sit down and eat will keep everyone on a healthy eating schedule, and allow you to plan your cooking schedule appropriately.

Speaking of snacking between meals, keep a lot of healthy snacks on hand. Everyone gets hungry sometimes and having healthy snack items available will ensure that you aren't ruining your healthy eating plans with snacks between your healthy meals. Keep a stock of nuts, dried fruit, fresh fruit, fresh vegetables, cheeses, and whole wheat crackers available to munch on when your stomach is feeling a bit empty. Planning healthy snacks ahead of time, and keeping them on stock, will make sure you never have an excuse to dig into a candy bar or bag of chips instead.

Healthy foods should be appealing. Even the pickiest of eaters can find a way to enjoy eating different kinds of good-for-you foods. For many kids display is everything. They may not want to eat fruit if they're just sitting on a plate. But if you arrange the fruits in a way that make them look like a rainbow (using strawberries for the red beam, oranges for the orange beam, grapes for the green beam, and so on) eating fruit will be fun and more like a game than a chore. Be open to serving foods in different ways. Vegetables don't need to merely be cooked or served raw.

They can be stir-fried, baked, and mixed into other meals. You can also hide vegetables in different foods. Puree some peas and mix them into your spaghetti sauce. Your children will get an extra dose of veggies without even realizing it. Puree spinach and mix it into meat loaf. Puree carrots and add them to chicken noodle soup stock. Hiding vegetables within different meals makes them easier for picky eaters to eat. And if YOU tend to have trouble gobbling up those good-for-you but very bland vegetables, you can do the same thing in your own meals. Hide healthy foods behind the taste and texture of other foods that you enjoy.

So many parents under-utilize seasonings when cooking for their family. But one of the easiest ways to make meats, fish, vegetables, and fruits taste even more appetizing is to season them. Don't be afraid to experiment with different spices and study up on seasoning tips and tricks. There's a reason that top culinary artists around the world season their foods heavily. It makes food taste better! And it will make food taste better, not just to you- but to your kids as well. Fresh herbs are another great way to add healthy, all-natural foods to your diet as well.

Cook It' Out

The easiest way to get excited about eating healthy? Start cooking! There's only one way you're going to get in the habit of creating easy, healthy meals for you and your family- and that's by practicing. Cook, cook, cook. The more you cook, the easier preparing and finishing meals will be. You'll learn what meals your family likes, which ones are easiest for you to make, and which ones you want to serve most often. Try new recipes, techniques, seasonings, and substitutes.

Cooking with your children is a fun family activity and a great way to get everyone involved in healthy cooking. Let your children help prepare different foods according to activities that are appropriate for their age. Toddlers can help stir things, while older children can help chop and mix things with a mixer. Teens can help with the oven and stovetop. Making cooking a family activity allows you to do less work, and teaches your children valuable lessons in cooking healthy.

Don't get discouraged. Not every recipe is going to turn out the way you thought it would. Things may not always be as good as you assumed they'd be. And your family members may not enjoy everything you cook. That's okay! A part of learning to cook healthy is trial and error. It's okay to not like things, and it's okay if things turn out wrong. Don't take one bad meal as a sign that you can't cook healthy. You can. Even the best of chefs have days- and meals that just don't turn out how they'd wished they would have. Keep cooking and don't fret too much when things go wrong. You'll eventually find meals that turn out amazing as well.

Pre-prepare as many meals as possible. If you don't work on weekends, try to take an hour or two each Sunday to prepare a few meals for the week in advance. In the busy-ness of the week many people will use the excuse of their tight schedules to grab unhealthy foods, rather than eating healthy meals. On the other hand, if you've prepped healthy meals in advanced you can conveniently cook good-for-you foods even when you don't have the time to prepare them all at that moment.

Homemade freezer meals can truly become your best friend. There are tons of meals that you can prepare in advance, freeze, and then cook and eat later in the week (or month!). Freezer meals are great for moms who work or have very busy schedules during the day. If you don't have time to prepare a meal from scratch when dinner arrives, making freezer meals in advance can help you keep your healthy eating meal plan on track. Simply make a few meals ahead of time, and then pull them out of the freezer and cook them as you need them.

If you tend to have a more laid back schedule in the morning, but get busier as the day goes on- crock pot meals can be very convenient for you. You can prepare the meal in the morning before your day gets started, and then let the crock pot do the work cooking the meal throughout the day. By the time dinner arrives a delicious healthy supper will be available for you and your family. The preparation happens in the morning, so you don't have to worry about fitting it into your busier schedule later in the day.

Make a point to just get into the kitchen and have fun. Grab an array of healthy foods and experiment. Just have fun cooking and using new and different foods in new and different ways. The best way to discover healthy meals that you love is to make an array of different healthy meals to try. Eating healthy shouldn't be a chore, and although it may require a bit more effort- you should be able to have fun preparing and trying all kinds of new and healthy foods.

Eating Healthy 24/7

There are often times that, as a mom, we lose sight of our healthy eating goals. It's natural to have times when you struggle to eat healthy.

On-The-Go

One of the most common issues many moms run into is simply being too busy to munch on healthy things. We can't carry fresh fruit with us wherever we go. Between school, sports events, extra curriculars, homework, and the dozens of other battles we face each day- it can be hard to stick to healthy eating. We sometimes reach out for unhealthy snacks when we're busy and our family is constantly on the go. It's easier to stop and grab McDonald's than a healthy option, right? Not necessarily. There are a lot of healthy on-the-go options for quick pick-me-ups throughout the day.

Mixed Nuts, Dried Fruits, and Veggie Chips
All three of these foods are shelf-stable, which means you can keep them in your purse, in your car, and in your diaper bag. They can be munched on anywhere at any time. Mixed nuts are packed with protein which will help make you feel full if you just need to cure that aching stomach. Dried fruits have that sweet kick that can help curb the cravings for candy and other sugary items. And veggie chips have a salty crunch that matches other potato chips- but they're often much healthier than their Dorito and Cheeto counterparts.

Granola Bars
Granola bars, especially protein bars, are a great quick filling snack that won't completely ruin your healthy eating goals. Look for ones that are made primarily of natural ingredients like oats, flaxseed, chia seed, dried fruits, raisins, and nuts. Protien bars are the best option, because protein helps you feel full and gives you an extra boost of energy to help you get through to the next meal.

Whole Wheat Crackers
If dinner is just an hour away, but your stomach is relentlessly reminding you that it needs food, a few whole wheat crackers can make a great snack. The carbs in grains give you a quick burst of energy and make you feel full, but only for a short time. Because of this whole wheat crackers are a great thing to snack on when you're only a short ways away from a main meal, but you desperately need something healthy to cure your munchies.

Pre-Made Salads
Tossing a Ceaser salad in a tupperware container before you go to work, so you can quickly grab it when you get home is a great way to prepare a healthy meal that you can take with you later on. If you often find yourself going to your children's sports events, or waiting around at different practices and extra curriculars, making salads in advance that you can take to these events will help you walk right past the concession stand without a second thought. If you're a little hungry during your child's soccer match that hot dog and bag of chips is going to sound really tempting. On the other hand, if you've brought a salad with you to munch on- you can cure your hunger in a light and healthy way that also leaves room for a healthy family dinner later on.

Deli Sandwiches
Although deli meats, cheeses, and breads do tend to be a bit more over-processed than other meats, cheeses, and breads- they're still a lot healthier than deep fried, greasy, and overly salted fast foods. If you're choosing between a fast food burger and french fries, or a deli sandwich- choose the sandwich. It won't leave you feeling nearly as bloated or heavy as the greasy food will, and it's much healthier for you.

While Traveling

It's so easy to lose sight of healthy eating goals while traveling. Between yummy hotel eating establishments, jet lag, and exhausting days of travel- taking a moment to be conscious about what you're putting in your body can be the last thing on your mind. On the other hand, continuing to eat healthy, even while traveling half-way across the country (or even half-way across the world) can be easier than you think.

Keep healthy snacks available in your hotel room.
Make a point to keep healthy snacks in your hotel room. Most hotel lobbies have small stores with snacks. Other larger resort lobbies may even have small grocery stores. Hotels in tourist-y areas are usually located near convenience stores with food options available as well. Search out the healthiest foods possible at these places. Nuts, whole grain breakfast cereals, fruit juice, yogurt, fresh fruit, and veggie chips are all good options. Keep a stock of these items available in your room throughout your stay. Even if you choose to eat unhealthy during a few big meals, if you continue to snack on healthy items throughout the day, you won't be eating nearly as horribly as you would be if you were eating unhealthy meals and unhealthy snacks.

Choose 'better' fast foods.
Yes- there are 'better' fast foods. Deli sandwich facilities like Quiznos and Subway tend to have better meal options than burger joints like McDonald's and Burger King. You can also choose healthier options at different fast food places. Breakfast yogurts and oatmeal instead of pancakes. Salads instead of fried chicken. Mixed fruit instead of french fries. Minimize your fast food consumption as much

as possible, but when you absolutely need a quick meal-choose the healthiest one possible.

Stay hydrated.
A common mistake that many people make when flying is that they tend to not drink enough. Flying causes you to get dehydrated, and dehydration makes you thirsty- and hungry. Yep, often times your body will mistake thirst for hunger. And you'll end up eating more than you usually would have, because you assume you're hungry, when in fact you're only thirsty. Make sure to drink plenty of water while you're traveling. Not only is it healthy for you, it will also help keep your hunger at bay.

Stick to at-home meal times.
When you're at home what time do you eat breakfast, lunch, and dinner each day? Try not to veer too far from your at-home schedule when you travel. If you continue to eat meals at the same times you do when you're home, your body will be able to stay on the same schedule- which will prevent you from feeling hungry at random times. It may take a couple days for your body to adjust its eating habits to the new time zone. Try to stick to eating at regular times, and if you need to snack- choose light healthy options. Regulating your body into a new time zone's eating schedule can help make your trip more enjoyable. Not only can it prevent constipation, bloating, and other digestive issues- it can help you stick to a healthy eating regimen and prevent overeating.

When You Eat Out

My personal biggest weakness when it comes to healthy eating is eating out.

Don't Use 'Dining Out' As An Excuse To Eat Poorly

I LOVE eating out. With that being said, I have this horrible habit of using eating out as an excuse to eat poorly. That's a really big 'no no'. When you decide to dine out with your partner, friends, or kids- keep your healthy eating plans in mind. Don't use eating out as an excuse to indulge yourself in an array of unhealthy foods. It's totally fine to treat yourself to a meal you typically wouldn't eat. On the other hand, it's not okay to order a big plate of greasy appetizers, a deep fried entrée with a salt-ridden side, and a sugar-filled dessert. Choose one meal that you really want to indulge in, and then opt to make the rest of your dining experience as healthy as possible. Don't use 'dining out' as an excuse to 'dine like crazy'.

Choose Healthier Establishments

There are certainly better restaurants than others out there. Chain restaurants like Olive Garden and Chili's tend to cook with over-processed, frozen foods. On the other hand small family-owned, and gourmet restaurants tend to opt for more natural, fresh, organic ingredients. A frozen, over-seasoned burger ridden with preservatives is a lot less healthy than a burger made with fresh ground beef, veggies, and cheese. Choose to eat at places where you know the food is fresh, not processed.

Start With A Salad And A Water

If you're eating at a place that offers salads before the main course, choose one. Eating a salad before you have your entrée can help control your hunger. It will fill you up on lighter foods, so when the heavier foods arrive you won't overindulge and spend the rest of the day feeling overly full. Also, making a point to drink a glass of water before your meal arrives can help tame your hunger and keep you from overeating.

Substitute Your Sides
Are you delving into a pretty calorie-ridden entrée? Maybe something like a fried chicken sandwich or a cheeseburger? In that case, try to find a healthier side. Instead of going for fries try something like a fruit salad or mashed potatoes. It's fine to eat fatty, greasy foods in moderation. But don't opt for making them your entire meal. If you really want fries, go for a lighter main course- like a grilled chicken breast. Whatever the case, try to only have one 'unhealthy' food on your plate at a time.

At The Office

Many of us work office jobs that require us to eat at least one meal while we're at our business. The hardest part of eating healthy for many individuals is eating at work. Convenience often rules over nutrition when you need a quick yet filling meal mid-way through the work day. Most of us will go to a fast food restaurant or pick up something that isn't necessarily super-healthy, but is convenient at the local convenience store. But for those of us determined to eat healthy in the office, all hope is not lost. There are a few little steps you can take to make a big impact on your lunch-time nutrition.

Use Their Refrigerator
Yes, that community fridge can totally be used by you. So quit ignoring the fact that it's there and start putting food in there. With that glorious cool-air filled container you can keep fresh fruits, veggies, deli meats, cheeses, and a variety of other healthy food options ready for your disposable. You're way more likely to munch on something natural and healthy when it's waiting for you in the rec room.

Budget Your Coffee Breaks
No, we get it. You definitely need that energy boost and coffee is a must. We're not telling you to quit drinking coffee, we're just saying that maybe you could slow down a bit. Coffee usually comes with creamers and sugars and lots of extra calories. Although it's a great appetite suppressant that can keep you from munching on other unhealthy foods, it still carries some unhealthy attributes. Try to budget yourself and if you notice that you're going back to the coffee machine multiple times a day- try to drink some water instead. It will trick your body into thinking you're full and help wean you off of that ever-addictive caffeine boost.

Bring Your Own Drink (Avoid The Vending Machine)
Speaking of water, bring a water bottle to work. That vending machine is filled with so many unhealthy yet tempting fizzy drinks. Ignore the temptation! Instead, bring your own water bottle and fill up on good ole H2O. You'll feel better, you'll be eating healthier, and you'll have an excuse not to spend $1.00 each day on a drink that isn't even good for you.

Granola Bars Can Be Your Best Friend
Yes- energy bars, protein bars, granola bars, whatever you want to call them; keep them in your desk! Dried fruit and nut mixes are great alternatives. Just keep something small and healthy to munch on when you're craving a snack. Reaching for a healthy snack from home instead of a bag of chips from the local convenience store is going to give you more energy and get you over that 3:00 PM hump in a healthier way.

Create A Food Budget
One of the best ways to motivate yourself to quit eating unhealthy is to start budgeting your grocery diet. Budget everything you eat. Factor in work meals, vending machine purchases, lunch breaks- everything. You'll be surprised how much you spend on expensive lattes and work-break snacks. Then you can start monitoring what you buy and finding better alternatives. You'll learn that bringing in that fruit from home (and using the work's fridge!!!) is way more affordable than going out and buying a sandwich for lunch every day. It's also way healthier.

Amidst a tough work day, taking the time to treat yourself to a healthier diet can give you more energy and keep you more attentive. Even the most technical of jobs get a little easier when you have a boost from a good hearty meal.

Now isn't that a good enough excuse to begin eating healthy at work?

During The Holidays

Let's face it, there is A LOT of delicious food available during the holidays and it's a time notorious for weight-gain. Call it modern American culture, call it a foodie's dream, call it whatever you want- it's a time when we're all bound to put on a few extra pounds if we're not careful. So what can we do? What precautions can we take to ensure our pants size stays the same even through the holiday season?

Eat On A Smaller Plate
Pick up a dessert plate rather than a dinner plate to serve yourself on. Because you cannot fit as much food on the plate, you won't feel obliged to eat as much food. If you're still hungry, get up for seconds. You're less likely to overeat when you're eating from a smaller plate. It also forces you to grab only the portion size you need. "Your eyes are bigger than your stomach" is true. And a smaller plate will help budget how much your eyes can take.

Wait 15 Minutes Before Getting Seconds
You often will not register as being 'full' for 15 minutes after eating a meal. So sit around, talk, laugh, drink some water for fifteen minutes after you've eaten. If you're still hungry, get up and grab more. If not, you just prevented yourself from overeating by waiting for your stomach to realize it was full before you filled your plate again.

Eat What You Love The Most
Many people try really hard during the holidays to eat healthy- only to end up 'giving up' and overindulging on everything. It's totally okay to let yourself eat what you want for a while. So look over everything that's being offered and find the 3 top foods you absolutely want to eat. Grab them, eat them. Then supplement the rest of your

plate with healthier options. You'll feel like you're indulging, but you'll be evening it out with healthier things on the side.

Don't Think You 'Need' To Try Everything
Which brings me to my next point- don't think you need to try everything. You don't. Once again, pick the things you really want to eat. Eat them. Don't pick up a serving of every casserole, cookie, and pie that's available. It all may look and smell delicious, but your body doesn't need that much food. Save the leftovers for later and focus on just eating the foods you absolutely want to eat, rather than trying everything you want to try.

There's a lot of temptation to over-eat and eat unhealthy during the holidays, but with a few guidelines you can definitely stay on track. Don't be afraid to indulge- just be cautious not to over-indulge.

Eating Organic on a Budget

Many people think that buying organic is expensive. Granted, some organic foods do have a bit higher of a price tag, but they actually aren't significantly more expensive than their pesticide-herbicide ridden counterparts. It's totally possible to buy organic on a budget, it's all about what you spend your money on and where you spend it.

Shop Local
Local farmer's markets and fairs are full of competitive prices and homegrown goodies. Buy in bulk from these small family-run farms and you're even more likely to

score some great prices. Creating personal relationships with local farmers can also get you some free goods. When they're overstocked and need to get rid of things before they go bad, you might be the special customer they have in mind to send their produce to. The food you buy from farmer's markets is also going to be significantly fresher than the options in the stores- which means it will probably have a longer shelf life. You won't have to use it as quickly, which means it's less likely to go bad and get thrown away.

Be aware of high-pesticide and low-pesticide fruits and veggies
Different foods within your supermarket are more likely to be ridden with pesticides than other foods. Know your 'low pesticide' and 'high pesticide' foods. Things like apples, strawberries, grapes, celery, spinach, and peaches are more likely to have a lot of pesticides on them. On the other hand, foods like mushrooms, avocados, sweet corn, pineapples, and cabbage tend to have very minimal pesticides.

Grow your own
When asked why people don't eat fresh foods many will say "I can't afford it" or "It's inconvenient" or "We don't have [insert name of edible plant] available at my grocery story". Excuses, excuses. Well you're not allowed to have those excuses anymore, because there are a ton of plants you can literally grow and eat right from your windowsill. The seeds and dirt will cost around $10.00 at most. And with a little water each day and a lot of sunshine, you'll have a healthy meal literally growing on your kitchen window.

Leaf Lettuce: One of the easiest, edible plants you can grow on your windowsill is loose-leaf lettuce. There are a variety of 'variety seed packets' for sale for as little as $0.99 USD. They'll grow hundreds of lettuce leaves and can quickly fill up a container. You can pluck them for salads, sandwiches, and any other recipe that requires lettuce. Once you snip them down, they'll also regrow multiple times- so you have a seemingly endless supply of fresh greens at your disposal.

Strawberries: Who doesn't love strawberries? These sweet little berries can be grow in containers in any south-facing window that gets a few hours of sun each day. They actually grow relatively easily and can even do well growing in the winter in cold climates (inside). Alpine strawberries are a small, but good beginner strawberry for indoor growers because they don't require much room but will get you a little harvest within 5 months or so.

Carrots: All you need to grow a carrot is a seed, some dirt, and a tall cup. Plant one seed in each cup and you'll have a carrot ready to harvest in about 70 days. Nutrired carrots are a great variety for growing indoors. They don't require a lot of care and are pretty tolerant to over and under watering, so even as a kids project you can usually have a fresh veggie ready to eat in a couple months.

Celery: Did you know you can take the bottom of your celery bundle and once all of the branches are removed, place it in water and allow it to take root? Then you can plant it in some dirt and new stalks with start to grow up. How resourceful! You won't be buying celery from the story anymore. All organic, hand-raised, and ready to be eaten right in your home.

Onions: Onions are slow growers, but once they're full grown they can be harvested, cleaned, and stored away in a cool cupboard for many months. They'll take about 6 months to mature on your windowsill, but if you plant the seed in a wide Tupperware container and let it grow in a partial-sun area, you'll have your own onions for your pantry in half a year's time.

Radishes: If you want some fresh food quick, radishes (and loose leaf lettuce- as mentioned earlier) are a great way to go. Radishes grow really REALLY fast. In fact you can probably harvest a full-grown radish from your windowsill in about a month. And just like carrots all they require is a tall cup and some dirt.

Garlic: Don't throw out those growing cloves in the back of your refrigerator. Plant them in some dirt with the white part entirely covered and the green stem sticking out. Water regularly and in a few months that one small clove will have grown into an entire piece of garlic that you can harvest and eat. (Just shhh- don't tell the grocery store owners about this. We're stealing their business with all these great ideas).

Leafy Herbs: Almost any loose leaf herb like Parsley, Basil, and Dillweed can be grown in a container on your windowsill. In fact there are many 'windowsill herb growing kits' available online and probably at your local gardening center. If you use dried herbs regularly, then you'll definitely want to look into growing your own. They're fresher and organic- so they have more vitamins and no preservatives or additives.

Black Pepper: Yes- you read that right. The most used seasoning in the world can be grown on your windowsill. Although this plant does best with more experienced growers that can get the right humidity and light requirements for it, it does provide you with awesome peppercorns that you can harvest and dry and use; the freshest pepper you'll probably every have.

Thought you didn't have any way to have fresh, organic, natural foods available near your home? Think again. This is just a small portion of plants that can literally be grown right in your home. With a bit of sunlight, water, dirt, and some seeds- you'll have your kitchen full of healthy plant-based foods in no time.

Emotional Eating

You had a bum day, things went bad, and you went into the kitchen to make yourself feel better. We've all done it at some point. Delved into the freezer, pulled out ice cream, and drown our sorrows with our stomach. We all know this habit is an unhealthy one, but sometimes it's a clutch that we rely on to get through tough times. Eating makes us feel better, so when we don't feel good- we reach out for food for comfort. But we don't have to eat to feel good. There are an array of ways to de-stress without eating, and you don't have to be a stressed-eater to forever.

Acknowledge When It Happens
They say the first step to healing is admitting that you have a problem. Stress eating is a real problem, and it's nothing to be ashamed of, but it's definitely something you need to acknowledge and admit is happening. So each time you pick up food when you're feeling emotionally upset, stop- and tell yourself what you're doing. It's hard to admit that you're not eating because you're hungry, but admitting that you're eating for the wrong reasons will help you avoid that behavior in the future.

Don't Make Excuses
The easiest way to continue to stress-eat is to make excuses when you eat. "Just this one time." "I deserve this." "I have

no other way of coping right now." are all common excuses we'll throw around when we pick up that bag of chips and eat the entire thing because we feel sorry for ourselves. The next time you make an excuse for as to why you're eating, stop yourself. Admit the real reason. And put the tub of ice cream down.

Write Down What You Eat, When You Eat It, and Why
Every day, for each meal you eat keep a food diary. Write down what you ate, when you ate it, and why. Were you actually hungry? Or were you bored? Or were you feeling sad and wanted to feel better with the help of a container of oreos? Be honest. Keeping track of what times you emotionally eat and what you grab to eat during those times will help you become aware of when you're emotional eating. If you tend to get stressed at work and eat unhealthy during your lunch break, and you've written that down every day- you know the exact time and place you need to work on changing your habits.

Set Goals To Change Your Ways
Once you've began keeping your food diary, analyze what you've learned and set goals to change your ways. If you tend to eat because of stress, try different ways of coping (meditate, try breathing exercises, get active, write down lists of what's bothering you). If you tend to eat when you're sad, try talking to friends and family about your emotions instead- or writing a diary to 'let things go'. And if you eat when you're mad, put your anger into a physical activity that will wear off calories instead of gaining them.

Always Ask Yourself "Am I Hungry?"
Before you sit down to eat something ask yourself "Am I hungry?" and then answer honestly. Are you truly hungry? How long has it been since you ate last? Do you still feel full? Are you just bored or is your body actually telling you

it needs food? Listen to your body's signals. You know when you're actually hungry and when you're not. Eat only when you're actually hungry.

Set Definite Meal Times and Meal Plans
Each day you should eat three balanced meals. Breakfast, lunch, and dinner. Small healthy snacks in between are totally fine. Plan out all three of your major meals (and any snack times) throughout the day. Set up recipes for what you will cook. And then, eat at those times every single day. Eat only what you've planned for yourself to eat. Don't reach out for something extra 'when you feel like it'. And if you're not actually hungry enough for that 3:00 PM snack, skip it. Focus on your three major meals each day, eat healthy, eat regularly- and stick to a schedule. Eventually your body will get in the habit of being fed at those times and stop feeling hungry at the signs of stress and other triggers that make you feel like you need to eat currently.

Keep Working Towards It
It's okay if you mess up a couple times. Bad habits are hard to break and you're not required to succeed the first time you try to stop stress eating. Just the fact that you admitted you have a problem and you're working to fix that problem has made you a success story. So don't get upset when you accidentally fall into old ways. Pick up the pieces and take it as a lesson learned. The more you break the habit, the less the habit controls your life. It'll be hard, but getting healthy is always worth it.

Eating Healthy Long-Term Tips

Becoming a life-long healthy eater is the best commitment you can make to your body and your health. But many people fall off track. They eat healthy for a while, and then they go back to bad habits- and eat unhealthy. They spend their life battling between the phases of eating well and eating crap. Eating well all the time shouldn't have to be an uphill battle. It should be an easy stroll. And there are a few different things you can do to make healthy eating an easier and happier habit to fall into.

Be An Adventurous Eater
Try new foods. Take a stroll down the produce aisle and pick up a fruit you've never tried before. Visit exotic grocery stores. Try different sea foods, meats, and dairy products from around the world. Be willing to take a taste of a variety of foods. You never know what new healthy and exciting food you'll fall in love with. The more healthy foods you try, the bigger your repertoire of healthy foods you love becomes. Don't limit yourself to only eating things you know you like. Try new foods often, and allow yourself to discover new foods that you may like equally as much.

Don't make the 'I ate unhealthy once- rest of the day' excuse
I am at fault of this. MANY of us are at fault of this. We'll eat one bad meal. Maybe we'll binge eat three donuts on our lunch break. And then we say to ourselves "Well, I should just eat unhealthy the rest of the day- because I just broke my 'healthy' streak by eating all of these donuts. I'll just start eating healthy again tomorrow. But, as for now, I'll just eat unhealthy the rest of the day." DON'T do this! There isn't even a legitimate argument behind this excuse. That's like saying, "Well I lost $20.00 gambling, I should just give the dealer the rest of the money in my wallet." It makes no sense. Don't eat unhealthy for the rest of the day, just because you ate unhealthy at one meal. You wouldn't

give all of your money to the dealer at the blackjack table just because you lost one game, would you? Of course not. So don't apply that same illogical idea to the way you eat. It's fine if you indulge. It's okay if you accidently eat one too many cookies. Forgive yourself and move on. But don't use it as an excuse as to why you should continue to let yourself eat unhealthily the rest of the day. That just doesn't make sense.

EXERCISING

Once you've mastered the art of putting healthy things into your body, you should have the energy and nutrients you need to starting behaving in a healthy way with your body; exercising. Exercise is an intimidating word to many people. It's often mistaken as this tough thing that involves lifting heavy weights and running five miles each day. To the contrary, all exercising really means is getting active. Working up a sweat doing activities- any activities. Exercising doesn't need to happen at a gym or with work-out equipment. It can literally happen anywhere, at any time. The first step to becoming a fit mom, is by finding a way to exercise that appeals to you. Some people enjoy going to gyms, lifting weights, or running five miles. If you're one of those people- great, do those things! But if you're not, that's okay. Find a way to get active that appeals to you.

That can be anything. It can be doing yoga with a yoga DVD instructional video in the comfort of your living room. It can be taking a bike ride with your dog. It can be taking a nature walk at your local park. Exercising can literally be anything that gets you up, off the couch, and moving. Find something you enjoy, and then- make a point to do it.

Make It A Habit

Just as though eating healthy is a habit that you need to develop, so is exercising regularly. The difference between eating and exercising is that you NEED to eat. Eventually you get very hungry and you have to eat. On the other hand, there's no physical necessity pushing you to exercise. That has to be done entirely by you. Your body isn't going to tell you when it needs to exercise. You have to decide that on your own, and you have to be the one to make the decision to get up and do it. You have to forcibly make it a habit.

Start by picking a time each day that works best for you. Some health experts will tell you that morning is the best time to exercise. Others will say your lunch break is an ideal time. The truth is- the best time to exercise is the time you choose to exercise. You know your body and your habits better than any health expert ever could. If you tend to get a burst of energy in the evening after work, then make a plan to exercise during that time. If you feel best in the morning, exercise in the morning. Choose a time that works best for YOU. One of the hardest parts of exercising is finding the time to get active. Many people opt to do it in the morning, before the day gets started. They knock that little goal off of their 'to do' list as soon as the sun comes up. Some of those people are naturally morning people, and for them- they're lucky. Because the rest of us are NOT morning people, and waking up and getting active can be really difficult. With that being said, there are a few things you can do each morning that will help boost your energy and get you moving at the crack of dawn.

Wake Up And Get Moving Immediately

Yes- the second your alarm gets off you need to get up and

do something. Anything. Don't lay around and allow yourself to slowly get up and get ready. Boosting your body into overdrive immediately will kick start your energy levels and get you motivated to go out and do something. So do some jumping jacks or squats or simply run in place for a minute. It's what you need to get up and get going.

Don't Hit The Snooze

Speaking of alarms, never hit the snooze button. Each time you allow yourself to fall back to sleep, you're exhausting your body's morning energy. So, as hard as it may be to pull yourself away from the cozy covers- do it. You're more likely to feel awake throughout the day if you get up the first time that buzzer goes off.

Have A Partner Ready To Get Up With You

Having someone to hold you accountable in your morning endeavors is going to make you more likely to wake up. So find someone to get up early with you. If you know someone else is counting on you to get out of bed, you're way less likely to make an excuse as to why you should sleep in instead. Even your dog can be a great morning buddy. If they're dying to go outside first thing when you wake up- you'll feel guilted into getting up, which will work to your advantage.

Drink Something Fruity

That citrusy sweet flavor of fruit stirs up your taste buds and gives you a secret energy boost. Even the smell of citrus is bound to get you up and moving. So opt for some fruit juice instead of caffeine in the morning. Caffeine will give you energy that will last a while, but fruit will get you started on an energy run that will get you through the whole day.

Shower In The Morning

A quick, cool shower can help awaken your senses. When you hop in the shower every part of your body's sensory receptors are on call- because they feel the water touching them. You're literally waking up your entire body at once, and by the time you're clean and ready to go, your energy level will definitely be higher. To the contrast, really hot showers can actually make you more tired by relaxing you. So opt for warm to luke-warm soaks instead.

Using Refreshing- Not Calming Scents When You Bathe

Speaking of bathing in the morning, did you know that the smell of your shampoo, conditioner, and body wash can actually have an effect on how well you wake up? Yep- it can. Calming scents like lavender and vanilla are more likely to keep you drowsy. On the other hand refreshing scents like melon and cucumber are more likely to have you feeling energized rather than relaxed when you leave the water.

Put On Music

Some nice, quick-beat music that you enjoy can boost your mood and definitely motivate you to get active. So don't be afraid to put on your head phones and turn up the volume. It'll help you get your day off with way more of a kick.

Leave Your House

Get up and go somewhere. Walk around your neighborhood, take your dog for a walk, go for a run, go to the gym- just leave the house. Simply being outside and seeing the sunshine for a moment, or changing environments can stir up your inner morning person. Who said seeing the sunrise wasn't worth it? No one- that's who. So get outside and find your chance to view it. You'll be surprised how much it wakes you up in the morning.

Waking up is hard- waking up and exercising first thing in the morning is harder. But starting off the day with that adrenaline rush can leave you with an energy and mood boost that will last the rest of the day. But getting active the second the sun comes up isn't required in order to get fit. For many mom's morning work-outs fit into their schedules. But if there's another time of day that works better for you, then by all means- exercise during that time. Find a time when you have energy and can dedicate 30 minutes each day to getting your heart pumping.

Write Down Your Goals

Writing down your fitness goals allows you to visualize them. You'll hold yourself accountable when you can see your goals staring right back at you. Hang them up on your bathroom mirror, on your fridge, near your keys- anywhere where you'll see them every day and can remind yourself that you -need- to do this. The guilt complex of constantly being reminded to exercise will help push you to actually get out and do it.

Get Active In Multiple Ways

Having an active lifestyle does not merely involve getting off the couch and exercising for thirty minutes a day. Being a fit person means that you make a commitment to being active as often as possible. You make physical activity a major part of your daily life. Getting your heart pumping becomes a second nature activity, because you've incorporated so many aspects of your day into your physical fitness activity.

Clean With Energy

One of the best ways to get active every single day? Make cleaning a physical fitness activity. Whether you're a mother to one child or five children, every mom out there knows that cleaning is just a fact of life for parents. You've already made cleaning a habit. Now, make it a fitness habit. But how? "Clean With Energy". There are a few different ways to accomplish this, but one of the easiest is to 'speed clean'. When you're cleaning in a hurry, you're moving quickly, building up a sweat, and yep- working out (while getting household tasks done- can you say win win?)! But there are a lot of other ways that you can make cleaning into a daily exercise regimen.

Vacuuming: Vacuums are heavy. Period. Pushing them back and forth works out your arms and abs. Lugging around that thing is a work out in and of itself (and if you're finishing a large room you've probably worked up a sweat by the time you're finished), but there are a few things you can do to push your body even further.

-Long, slow, pushes back and forth: Because vacuums are fairly heavy, pushing them slowly in long strokes back and forth will work out your arm muscles even more than it would if you were doing quick pushes. Make sure to extend your arm all the way for each push, and pull the vacuum as far back to you as possible when you're drawing it back in.

-Switch arms regularly: To get a full workout, switch your

arms regularly throughout the time you're vacuuming. Vacuum one room with your right arm, and the next with your left. Or you could even change them up between pushes. Just make sure you're not focusing all of your energy and efforts into one arm.

-Lunge with each push: Want to get your legs working as well? With each long push you make with the vacuum lunge forward on one foot. Match the foot to your arm (if you're pushing with your right arm, move your right foot forward) bend your knee down and lunge. Push back up, and as you bring the vacuum back to you, stand back into a straight position.

-Lift the vacuum between rooms rather than rolling it. Vacuums are practically free weight-lifting equipment. Rather than rolling or dragging them between rooms, pick them up and carry them. It's way more work, and it's way more physical activity.

Sweeping/ Mopping: Start by clearing as many rooms in your house as possible. The more floors you can clean at once, the longer and more strenuous your 'sweep and mop' work out will be.

-Fast quick strokes: Unlike a vacuum, brooms and mops are relatively light-weight, so long slow strokes with them won't necessarily get you a great work out. On the other hand, fast strokes will- because it will get your body moving. Try to mop and sweep as quickly as possible to get a good heart-pumping workout in.

-Hand-wash in a push-up position: If you need to hand-scrub a few parts of your floor, rather than simply sitting on your hands and knees, try scrubbing the floor in a push-up position. Not quite strong enough to hold yourself up? Put your knees down and do a 'girl's push up' instead. It will help work your arms and abs while making your floors sparkling clean.

Dusting: Dusting is a common household chore that doesn't usually require a lot of effort. With that being said, it can turn into quite a work-out if you go into it with the right attitude.

-Squat to reach lower areas: Don't bend down to reach lower areas, instead work out those legs and butt with a squat. Each time you need to reach a lower area to dust, spread your feet apart, shoulder's width from one another. Then bend your knees down and squat to reach the area.

-Jog in place: While you focus on dusting different meticulous places around the house, try jogging in place to get your heart racing. You can also jog between the areas you need to dust.

-Do windows and mirrors regularly: Mirrors and windows can become your new best friend. Those tall, lengthy surfaces are the perfect place to focus on. All of that reaching and long pushes of your arm muscles will pay off in a raised heartbeat.

-Use vertical strokes on windows and mirrors: Speaking of windows and mirrors, when you do focus your time on them- use vertical strokes. They're harder than horizontal strokes. You'll be forcing yourself to push up and down (against gravity) with each dusting swipe. Your biceps will thank you for it later.

-Wax on, Wax off countertops: When you get to your counter tops, use two rags- one in each hand, and focus on doing circular motions. Have a wet rag in one hand and wipe one portion of the counter clean. Have a dry rag in the other hand, and dry the same portion of the countertop before moving to the next spot. This will work out both of your arms and the circular motion takes more effort (and gets a more thorough clean) than a simple back and forth movement.

Folding Laundry: Laundry and dishes are the two chores that are required to be finished almost daily. Somehow, the washer and dryer are endlessly full. Luckily for you, that stack of clothes is an opportunity to get active.

-Put clothes in the washer/ dryer one at a time- but quickly: When you are moving clothes from the hamper to the washer, bring one item of clothing to the washer at once. But, move the items as quickly as possible. It will force you to work harder moving all of the clothes from one area to another, and the quick movement will get your blood pumping. You can copy the same idea when you move the clothes from the washer to the dryer as well.

-Move clothes from dryer to basket, but place basket on top of dryer: If you have a front facing dryer, place the basket on top of the dryer rather than in front if it when you are taking the clothes out of the dryer. You'll have to move the clothes up to the basket, which will be a bit more work and help your abs and arms get a small work-out as you empty the dryer.

-Do wall-sits: While folding clothes, try doing periodic wall sits. Place your back against the wall and bend your knees until you are in a sitting position. Balance against the wall while you fold the clothes. Your legs will be toned in no time.

-Take clothes to rooms individually rather than in a basket: For each member of the family, take their stack of clothes to their room individually. Rather than carrying all of the clothes in one basket, you'll be walking back and forth, getting in more exercise in the process. Want to up the cardio? Try jogging each set of clothes to each room.

Making The Bed: Probably the first chore of the day, making the bed is a quick task. There isn't a lot you can do to make this work any more strenuous, but there are a few things you can try that will get your heart racing a bit faster.

-Flip the mattress weekly: It's a lot of work, yes. But if you want to throw in an extra activity to keep your mattress in top condition and get you worked into a fitness mode- try flipping the mattress yourself. You'll work out practically every muscle of your body, and your mattress will stay in better shape, longer.

-Time yourself: Make the bed in a speedy way. Tuck in that sheet, spread out that cover, and place those pillows perfectly on the bed as quickly as possible. You'll get the chore done faster, and your heart pumping faster.

Washing Dishes: Just as with laundry, washing dishes can be a great opportunity to get your heart pumping. Although sitting and scrubbing plates and bowls may seem like a stationary activity, it can actually turn into quite a work-out with the right goals in mind.

-Hand wash, rinse, and dry: If you have the time, even if you have a dishwasher, hand washing even a portion of your dishes can help you get moving. You'll be standing, and moving your arms- which although it may not seem like much, will ultimately burn more calories than sitting on the couch while the dishwasher does all the work.

-Do calf raises: A great exercise to do while you're washing dishes is calf raises. Start by spreading your feet slightly apart and then raising your heels off of the floor (standing on your tippy toes). Hold for ten to fifteen seconds and then slowly sit your feet down. Repeat the exercise to help tone your calves.

-Put away dishes one by one, quickly: This idea mimics the same exercise we mentioned with the laundry. Rather than grabbing a lot of the dishes and putting them all away at once, grab each dish individually and put it away as quickly as possible. It will force you to move faster as you clear all of the dishes out of the rack.

Cleaning Up (Misc): Between clothes, shoes, toys, and other household objects that manage to get moved out of place throughout the day- mom's are inevitably always cleaning up... stuff. Welp, turn that 'stuff' into your personal workout motivation. Because cleaning up, can definitely be a get-fit activity.

-Squat to pick up each individual item off the floor: Just as with dusting, rather than merely bending down to reach something at a lower level, squat. Your legs and butt will thank you for it in the long run. And depending on the amount of toys, homework, or random clothes scattered all over your house- you may get in a good set of squats each day without even realizing it.

-Speed walk items back to original room: Don't leisurely walk each item back to its original room. Instead, speed walk them there. You're moving faster, and in so- being more active. Speed walk as often as possible as you do different chores and pick up different items.

-Speed-scrub the showers: And lastly, don't forget the bathroom! There are a lot of places you can scrub down in there, but one of the best ones to get a work out on is the shower. Speed-clean that shower as quickly as possible. Scrub it down and time yourself while you do it. The quick movements as you have to move your body from very high to very low places will work up a sweat in no time.

While Pregnant

Many women out there take pregnancy as a sign that they shouldn't exercise at all. They should be focusing on keeping their body safe from injury, and because of this many moms completely opt out of exercise during pregnancy. With that being said, exercising during pregnancy is beneficial to both you and your baby. It can help regulate your digestive system, circulatory system, balance, and help with preventing typical aches and pains that coincide with growing a baby. Pregnant women should exercise with caution. Avoid any high-energy activities. Any high-impact activity like volleyball, football, or basketball typically aren't the best options. Any activity where you are bouncing, running, or could fall (like bicycling or rock climbing) are also best left for non-pregnant moments. Instead, focus on low-strenuous activities. Find physical fitness techniques that you can do without putting too much stress on your body. Yoga: Yoga's slow pace and focus on centering of the body and mind can be beneficial to many pregnant women. The controlled breathing practice can help you during labor, and yoga's focus on muscle strength and flexibility is a great way to stay fit during all nine months of your pregnancy. You don't need to go fast paced and as your body changes you can find different positions and exercises that are comfortable and appropriate for your current trimester. Light Lifting: Want to keep those arms toned? Lifting light weights (2 to 5 pounds) during your pregnancy is safe and can help you work up a sweat and keep those arms strong and in shape. Other arm work-outs like bench presses and push-ups are nearly impossible with a baby belly (and not always safe with a baby belly). Opt for using light bar-bell style weight and pushing your muscles with slow, deliberate movements.

Flexibility/ Stretching

To keep your muscles and body in tip-top shape you should exercise as often as possible, but you should regularly have days where you take a break and focus on lighter activities. Stretching during these 'off days' is a great way to continue to focus on physical fitness without wearing your body down. Focus on your shoulders, chest, waist, and legs to help keep your body center aligned, even as everything rearranges with in you.

Walk, walk, walk

Walking is by far one of the best ways to get active when you're pregnant. Speed walking, walking on a treadmill, walking in parks and outside, and just generally walking around. Get up and get your blood moving. Try to walk for 15 to 20 minutes a day. You don't need to move fast, it's just about getting up and forcing yourself to be active.

Just keep swimming

To quote one of my favorite little fish (Dora from Finding Nemo), "Just keep swimming". Water arobics, swimming laps, and simply treading water are all great ways to raise your heartbeat with a baby in your belly. Practically any swimming sport (aside from diving) is safe for pregnant women, and they are one of the most highly recommended ways to stay active while pregnant by many doctors. There is a very low risk for injury, low strain on your muscles, and allow you to stay active without the risk of losing your balance or hurting yourself.

Stationary biking

Addicted to the gym, but not the biggest fan of the treadmill? Not all gym equipment is appropriate for pregnant women due to the odd angles and strain they can put on your body. With that being said, stationary bikes are a fantastic way to work out. Don't let your gym membership go to waste. Stationary cycling is a great way to burn energy and stay active, safely, while pregnant.

It's important to focus on your comfort and health, especially when exercising while pregnant. Do not put your child at risk. If something doesn't feel 'right', stop what you're doing. If you are in pain, your body changes temperatures, you have a rapid heartbeat, are finding it hard to breathe, or are facing any other abnormal symptom- do not continue to do what you are doing. Stop, and if the problem worsens, visit a doctor.

Remember to stay hydrated! Drink lots of water before, during, and after you exercise to ensure that you stay in tip top shape. Dehydration is bad for you and your child, so make sure you're getting enough water each day to sustain your daily activity and the sweat you are losing while you exercise.

Wear a very supportive bra. Those girls are growing right beside your belly. They need extra support during your pregnancy. Buy a maternity bra that fits, is comfortable, and supports your breasts appropriately. Visiting a place that can help you fit a bra correctly and find a personalized option for you can help guarantee that you're wearing the right size.

Skip the skin-tight clothes while you're pregnant and

exercising. Instead opt for loose-fitting comfortable clothing that will allow you to sweat and move comfortably. You want the best mobility possible, and tight constricting clothes won't allow you to do that. Although a baggy t-shirt and loose-fitting shorts may not be the most stylish outfit at the gym, it will certainly be the most functional.

Exercising while pregnant can be a challenge. There is a lot happening within your body that can make movement and fitness activities difficult. But making an effort to get active every single day can greatly benefit your body, and the little body growing inside of you. The easiest way to exercise while carrying a child is to maintain the habit right from the beginning. Don't stop exercising once you realize you're pregnant. Alter your exercises to be appropriate for your pregnancy, but don't discontinue exercising altogether. Continue to stay on track with fitness goals and your habitual daily physical activities. The sooner you make it into a habit, the easier it will be to maintain physical fitness activity throughout all three trimesters.

With A Baby

Ahh, the joys of having a baby. Between midnight feedings, diaper changes, and doctor's appointments, how in the world does a mom of an infant find time to exercise? It can be hard at times, but it isn't nearly as impossible as you think. In fact, many of the daily activities you do with your little one are already helping your body heal and rebuild itself after pregnancy and labor. One of the best ways to get your body back into tip top shape? Breastfeeding. Not only is breastfeeding fantastic for your child's health, it helps your body get back into the shape it was pre-pregnancy by burning an immense amount of body fat to produce the milk. Each time your little one fills their belly, you lose a bit of your belly fat. Your body is working overtime to produce the nutrients your child needs to grow big and strong, and it's pulling many of those nutrients away from the fat you've stored on your body throughout your pregnancy. So if possible, breastfeed your baby. It's the quickest way to kick start your body into getting back to its original physique.

Carry your little on around as often as possible. The skin to skin contact will soothe your baby and help them develop a strong emotional bond to you and the rest of the world. But, carrying your little one as often as possible also is a work-out. That little child can feel really heavy when you've been holding them the entire day. With newborns you can carry them in a front wrap carrier that will safely keep them close to you as you walk around. As your baby ages you can move onto other front and back carriers. Keeping your little one in toe as you do housework and basic chores will add to your muscle's workout. You'll essentially be getting more of a work-out while bonding with your baby. Win win, right?

Strollers are your new best friend! Once your child reaches around two months of age, you can safely begin strolling them around. Visit the mall, the park, or just walk around the block. Pushing a stroller around is a great way to get daily exercise while caring for your baby. Jogging strollers are another fantastic way to get active. They safely allow your child to be strolled at higher speeds while you jog behind. If you enjoy running, a jogging stroller is a great physical fitness investment.

Speaking of getting out with your little one. You can use a stroller or a carrier to bring your child on a hike. Hikes aren't typically done on as easy of terrain as a sidewalk, but with the right stroller (or a baby carrier) you and your little one can have a great adventure through a local nature area. The tougher terrain will be a more strenuous work-out, so even if you're going slow you'll still be pushing your body, burning calories, and building muscle.

While out and about with your little one, remember to be prepared. Bring a diaper bag with all of the basics including bottles, diapers, extra clothes, snacks and water for you, and basic first aid equipment for each of you. The more prepared you are, the less likely you are to end your exercise session early to run home and fix a problem that arose along the way. Bring what you need and carry it in a backpack or in a space under your stroller. You won't be able to make the excuse to go home and quit exercising for the day, if you can handle issues as they arise because you have what you need to deal with them on hand.

There are quite a few different strength exercises you can do throughout the day with your child without needing to pre-plan or put a lot of effort into them.

Front-Carry Squats
If you have your child held in a front carry wrap or carrier, try standing and doing squats while your child is with you. The extra weight will push your leg and butt muscles even further and help you get toned up fast.

Play Mat Push-Ups
Does your little one enjoy rolling around on their play mat. Rather than simply sitting with them, get in a push-up position and watch your little one play as you do a few

push-ups beside them. Not only will you be building upper body strength, you'll also be setting an example for them to learn how to push themselves up as well.

There are many different places including different swimming lessons, yoga sessions, and daycares that offer 'Baby n' Me' workouts. Essentially these are work outs created specifically for moms (and dads) and their babies. Signing up for one of these and attending them as regularly as possible are a great way to get active with your little one. Not only will you be getting some much needed exercise, you'll be creating a healthy exercise habit for your little one starting in their early years.

If you aren't quite ready to face the hiking trails, stroller walks, or mom n' me workouts, working out at home is a great alternative. If you have the funds you can purchase some at-home work-out equipment. If not, there are tons of great online work-out tutorials, exercise books, and DVDs that can inspire you to get up and get moving right from the comfort of your living rooms. Find one that appeals to you and find a time each day that you can dedicate to getting your heart pumping. When your little one is napping or playing, you can be getting in that necessary 30 minutes of exercise that your body needs to leave you feeling fantastic the rest of the day.

And lastly- don't forget to rest. When you have the busy-ness in your life that is a newborn, working out isn't your top priority. Although you should do it when you have the time and energy, rest is way more important at this stage in your little one's life. Make sure your body is getting enough sleep. Nap often, it's healthy for you- and your muscles, and your body in general. Your mind will feel better. So make sure you're getting your rest!

With Toddlers

What fun- the terrible twos and thrilling threes. We all love toddlers, but ugh- they sure do wear us out, don't they? Luckily for you, all of their energy can be a great motivator for your physical fitness goals. It's easy to get active when you have a kiddo who's equally as active and wants to be energetic with you. There are so many awesome ways you can get active with your little one. Exercise will be a breeze when you have a toddler in the home.

Goal number one: Make a point to wear them out each day. By the time bedtime comes around your little tike should be ready to hit the sheets. Whether you're a stay-at-home mom or a working mother, just taking an hour or two to get truly involved in your toddlers life can get you active and them actively worn out. It will benefit their little bodies and your body as well. Do things with your kiddo. Find fun things to do throughout the day and make a point to share them with your child.

Go outside.
Get outdoors with your little one. Whether you need to bundle them up for a winter romp in the snow or just throw on a pair of shorts and explore in some summertime weather, letting your little one roam in nature is a great way to boost your mind and body. Your toddler will have so many amazing sensory experiences, and chasing them around as they discover so many new things will keep you on your toes- which will help you burn some extra calories. So let them venture through the local park, play in the backyard, or build a snowman on the sidewalk. You'll be making memories and getting in exercise without even realizing it.

Go out to family activities.
Every city has family activities available for moms with toddlers. Whether it's a kid's day at the local museum, an event at the park, or a special occasion at the mall- bring your toddler along. It'll be a great moment for you to get in some socialization with other moms in the area, and your little one will have fun experiencing so many new things. Along with that, most of these events are catered to kids- which means they are high energy and have lots of opportunities for games and activities that involve both your little one and you to be up and moving.

Swimming Lessons.
Swimming lessons are a fantastic way to get active with your child. You'll be teaching them a valuable skill while also burning energy. Between treading water, kicking, and learning different strokes with your kiddo, you'll both be getting a ton of much needed exercise.

Kiddie Sports
Between t-ball, soccer, and golf there are many different opportunities for little kids sports out there. Volunteer as a coach (or just an involved parent) and let your little one try out some different sports. Running around with a group of toddlers is sure to wear out even the most fit adult, so getting involved with teams of little ones can be a great way to get yourself into shape.

Physical activities.
Just as with kiddie sports there are a ton of different physical activity opportunities for toddlers. Karate and ballet are two of the most popular and widespread opportunities for little ones. Typically, with toddlers, parents will be very involved in the lessons. You'll be on your feet and jogging around with your kiddo as well,

which will help you get in some extra exercise while your kiddo learns a new skill.

Chase em' around. At the end of the day, toddlers just have a ton of energy- and that's awesome. Chase them around. Keep them out of trouble. Play tag, hide n' go seek, and let them roam free while you keep a close walk behind. With the amount of energy toddlers have, just keeping close tabs on them is sure to wear you out. Stay on your feet. Be an involved and active mom, and exercise will be second nature through your kid's younger years. You'll be worn out just keeping up with them.

With Elementary Aged Kids

Elementary aged children can be a lot of fun to exercise with. With their energetic demeanors and yearning to be involved with their parents in activities, they're usually pretty easy to coax into some family bonding physical activity time. It's very healthy for them, and it can be a lot of fun for all of you. There are a lot of ways to get involved actively with your children.

If your child is interested in being involved in different sports, volunteer to be the couch (or help the couch out). You'll have the opportunity to teach a group of kids valuable lessons in teamwork and good sportsmanship. You'll also have the chance to do different warm up exercises with the kids, and be involved in their running, jumping, and playing. It's easy to get work-out when you're jogging with children back and forth across a field or court. And the best part of all is that you'll be able to be involved in one of your child's extra curriculars in a meaningful way.

Go to local family events and activities. Fairs, festivals, and children's days at different facilities around town can be a great way to get up and active as a family. Simply walking around different areas can get you more exercise than you'd get sitting at home watching TV. Plus, giving your child the opportunity to explore their hometown and meet other local children is a great social and educational opportunity for them. Whenever there are family events on days when you have nothing else to do, get off the couch and go. You'll have a chance to have fun as a family, and you'll probably be doing way more physical activity than you would be if you stayed home.

Get out and exercise as a family. There are a lot of ways you can make a point to do physical things with your kids each day. Pick an activity and make a habit of doing it each and every day. Take a walk around the block (or walk to the grocery store rather than drive). Grab an umbrella if it's raining (don't use weather as an excuse), and if the sun is shining- get out too. Take a walk around the block with your kiddos. It'll give you a chance to have some valuable talking time while you get those legs moving. Make a point to walk instead of drive when possible. If your grocery store, Post Office, or school is within walking distance- use those feet instead of your car. You'll save gas and money, while spending extra calories. Pick up your kiddos from school and walk them home each day. Just make a habit of using your legs instead of your vehicle when possible. It'll give your kids a chance to wear off some energy, and you an extra chance to get active throughout the day.

Explore your backyard or a local park.
Getting outside with your kid is not only a great way to get physically active, but it can be a great educational opportunity as well. Your child will have the chance to learn a lot of hands-on things about plants, animals, and the

eco-system around their home. There are an array of things you can do outside. Garden, go bird watching, go for a hike, build a tree house, go camping, go fishing, track animal prints in the snow, play in the snow, just get outside and make a point to discover things together.

Go to the local playground together.
Many mom's stand aside while their children wear off some energy at the local playground, but the playground can be a great place for you to get physically active as well. Push your child on the swing, run beside them as they slide down the slide, show them your talents on the monkey bars, play tag- just be genuinely involved in the activities your child is doing at the playground. You'll have a chance to be the 'fun parent' and an active parent. You won't even realize how much exercise you're getting in amidst all of the fun you're having.

Take a bike ride.
A daily bike ride can be a great activity for you and your child. Bike riding works out an array of muscles while also acting as a great cardio activity. You're moving your legs, raising your heart rate, using your arm muscles and ab muscles, and getting a good dose of fresh air. There are so many ways bike riding can benefit you and your child. It's a great activity to share with your family that many kids really do enjoy. So when your child gets a new bike, buy yourself one too- and make riding them into a family activity.

Swim.
Live next to a beach or a pool- or even have your own pool (even if it's just a kiddie pool)? Swim! Many kids love the water and when the weather gets hot you probably do to. So hop in, splash around, play with your children in the water.

With Teens

Teens can be either the hardest or easiest kids to get active with. They've grown to a point where physically, they are on the same level as you. They can run as fast as you, they can work out on the same equipment as you, they can play sports beside you in a competitive manner, and they can keep up with your pace in physical activities. They're young adults, and they can make fantastic exercise companions. With that being said, all teens don't love exercise. Creating a love of fitness does start at a young age, and as your child grows older it's harder to get them into the habit. They really need to make the decision on their own. You can inspire them, by offering to do activities that they enjoy- but at the end of the day living a physically fit lifestyle has to be their choice. Forcing your child to exercise will only make them hate exercising. Don't make it a consequence or a requirement. Make it a fun activity that you can do and enjoy as a family.

If your child is interested in exercising with you and wants to get physically fit alongside you, create an exercise plan together. In fact, when your child grows into a teen they can also begin to create fitness goals as we talked about in the first chapter (with goals set for each day, week, and month in advance). Set goals with one another for the activities you want to complete each day, week, and month. Maybe you both have the goal to work up to running 2 miles a day. Start small. Set the goal that at first you'll run ¼ a mile, and then ½ a mile- working up to 1 mile, 1 ½ miles, and ultimately two miles over a three to four month time period. Take things slow, but set goals together. Working with your teen to achieve different physical fitness activities can be a great way to keep you both motivated.

Is your child involved in any sports or extra curriculars? Help them practice. Whether it's ballet or basketball, you can find a way to be involved in helping your child master their activity. If they need a partner to practice with, be there- any time you can to help them practice. Offer to help them practice. Coach, attend practices, be involved in their team or club as often as you can. Let your child know that you are proud of their physical activity and you want to help them in any way possible. Don't push them- don't force them to do more than they can. But support them, and help them better themselves. At the same time, you'll also be getting active and showing your child that you can also be involved in the activities they enjoy and are passionate about.

Make a habit of getting out together and being active. Whether it's taking your dog walk, going for a bike ride, taking hikes, or going to the beach together- find ways to be active with one another each day. Little things do add up, and even a stroll around the block with your family pet can get both of you up and moving. It will boost your moods, give you a chance to spend some quality time with one another, and of course- get you active.

Choose high-energy family activities. Do you like to travel or get out and do things with your children? Choose to invest your time and money in things that will get you off of your feet. Rather than going to a movie, go play miniature golf. Instead of relaxing on the beach, take surfing lessons. Replace low-energy activities with things that are going to get you moving together. When you go on vacation choose to do activities like snorkeling, nature hikes, and ski'ing. When you're searching for things to do around your hometown find places that do activities like laser tag, rock climbing, and swimming. Everyone loves doing things together as a family, but when you have teens being active together can be one of the most fun ways to spend a day. Because they're on the same physical level as you- they can keep up with you and go at an adult pace. They can do more advanced activities than they could when they were younger, and they can be a part of a lot of adult experiences that you couldn't bring them along on when they were a child.

With A Tight Schedule

Some of us are busy- really really busy. We overbook ourselves to the point of exhaustion and on top of that we're required to eat healthy and be active? Impossible! How can anyone ever manage more things on top of an already full day of work and activities. We gotta sleep, right? Being active amidst being busy may be way easier than you think it is. You don't necessarily have to make time to go to the gym. There are plenty of ways to get fit just doing what you do- even when your calendar is totally booked up.

Be Active At Opportune Moments Rather Than Scheduled Ones
You don't need to make time to be active, you just need to acknowledge times when you can be active. If you're going grocery shopping, make an exercise out of it by speed walking. When you're at your child's sporting event opt to stand instead of sit (do squats against the wall and you're working even harder). Jog in place while you watch TV. Stretch while you're sitting down at the desk at your office. Walk to your lunch spot rather than drive. Find random moments throughout the day when you can be active and then take advantage of them.

Don't Over-Exhaust Yourself
One issue many people find when over-booking their schedules is that they are exhausted all of the time. Budgeting your time for the projects that are most important is a necessity in staying healthy and fit. No matter how busy you are, if you are too tired to accomplish tasks in a quality and efficient manner, you're not going to get things done as well or as quickly as you'd like. So rather than filling your schedule with everything you need to get done- find a way to focus on the most important activities and work hard on them. You'll have more energy, and in doing so probably be naturally more active as you accomplish daily tasks. You can always get to the smaller, less-important jobs eventually. So focus on the big ones and deal with the smaller ones as you have time and energy.

When You Have Spare Time, Use It To Be Active
Even the busiest of schedules have a couple moments of peace and quiet. Rather than using those moments to simply watch TV, try being active. And yes- you can totally watch TV while being active. Do jumping jacks, run in place, do yoga, or squats. There are literally hundreds of different activities you can do with just 5 spare minutes, no equipment, and right in the middle of your living room.

Keep A List Of Your 'Active Moments' Throughout The Day
When you do get a chance to exercise at a random moment, write it down. Have a goal to complete just ten 5 minute work-outs a day. You can space them throughout your schedule. You don't need to break a sweat, just get your heart rate up for a second. Ten, five minute work outs equals 50 minutes total. That's almost an hour of activity that you got throughout the day- in little jolts when you had time. And if you write them down you can keep track and

stay motivated. You'll constantly be looking for ways to get active so you can mark one more 'burst of exercise' off your list.

Realize That It's Okay If You Miss A Day- Or Two
If you are totally inactive and glued to your desk for the entire day, don't beat yourself up over it. It's totally okay to miss a day or two of forcing yourself to be active. Don't let a couple days of slacking make you a life-long slacker. Pick right back up where you left off. You don't need to exercise every single day in order to be successful. Try to exercise every day, but don't fret if you miss a couple. You can always start again.

If you're a working mom, staying active with a busy schedule can seem really hard- especially if you work in an office. Some of the best jobs in the world happen to be desk jobs. Jobs that require you to sit down at a desk. The most immobile thing you can do for 8 hours a day- and it's your job to do it. That doesn't mean your job isn't hard work, it just means you're most likely not that active while you're at work. But that doesn't mean you don't *have* to be inactive if you don't want to be. There are plenty of ways to start wearing off some energy and even exercising amidst a stay-still office job.

Walk During Your Lunch Break
If you tend to finish meals relatively quickly, try walking during your lunch break when you have extra time. Even a quick stroll around the office building can get your blood pumping enough to make it worth it. 15 minutes walking around your business's part of town is 15 minutes you weren't sitting still at your desk during the day. So when you get the chance to walk, take it.

Replace Your Chair With An Exercise Ball
I realize not all offices will allow you to do this, but if yours is open to it- try replacing your office chair with an exercise ball. Yes- one of those giant blue balls that you sit on. It will help with your posture and work out your abs, legs, and balance the entire time you're sitting on it. Plus, it's fun- so much more fun than sitting in a boring office chair.

Get Small Dumbbells And Lift Them
Keep small weights under your desk and during conference calls or tasks that don't require your hands, pick em' up and start lifting. This is one exercise you can literally do at any point throughout the day, even while sitting down. You may look a little odd, but what are the chances of someone seeing you in your cubicle anyways? And you might even start a fad around the office- a getting fit fad.

Stretch When You Get A Chance
Stretching promotes good circulatory function, it decreases stress, and it helps create muscle strength. Even while sitting in an office chair you can stretch your body in different ways. It's easiest to focus on your arms and back while sitting down. But you can even make a point to stretch your legs each time you get up. Working on your flexibility may not seem like the most efficient way to stay in shape, but it definitely helps your body's ability to work out. It's one small task you can do throughout the day at an office job that will benefit you when you're actually up being physical.

Speed Walk To Different Meetings And Breaks
Act like you're in a hurry. Who's going to know the difference anyways? For all they know you're late everywhere you go and have to walk fast to get there on time. But, you're actually just speed walking... well, to

speed walk. Speed walking gets your heart rate up and gets you moving just fast enough to have all of those muscles pumping. So speed walk to the bathroom, to the coffee machine, to the meeting down the hall.

Desk jobs are pretty widely recognized as being careers that require you to sit down and stay still. But you don't have to fall into that stereotype. There are definitely ways that you can be physically active in the work space if you make a point to get yourself into a get-fit mode every day.

Have A Friend or Partner

Why have an exercise partner?

Many personal trainers will swear that the reason their job makes other people successful is the fact that having someone to exercise with is more likely to keep you in shape. Whether or not you have a personal trainer doesn't matter. What matters is that you have someone beside you to be there with you as you work on your physical fitness endeavors. Just having someone else around can benefit you greatly in your chances of success.

They Hold You Accountable

Having someone waiting on you to exercise with them is one of the best motivators to get out and get active. If you know you have someone relying on you to get fit with them, you're way less likely to make excuses and skip out on getting out. When you have an exercise partner long gone are the days of "I'll just start tomorrow", because they're relying on you starting today.

They Are Your Physical Guilt Complex

And when you do miss a day of physical activity, your partner will be a visual reminder that you missed out. They'll be your walking guilt complex. If you missed out while they were active, you'll have more of a push to keep up with them in the future. No one wants to be left behind. And you definitely won't want to be sitting on the couch when your running partner is out there getting in shape.

They Keep You Company

Sometimes one of the most difficult parts of exercising is simply having no company while you work out. It's way more fun to have someone to chat with while you run, or just to run silently beside you. It's also less intimidating to visit a gym or try a new class when you have a friend beside you ready to help you if you need it.

You Can Do Duo Workouts- Or Singular Ones, Together

When you have a partner exercising with you, you open up more fitness activities for yourself. You can do two-person exercises that require a friend or a 'spotter' to accomplish. You can also play two person sports like tennis and racket ball. They make one person sports like golfing and biking more fun. And they're there beside you during your 'one man workouts' just to keep you company while you both get active, together.

They Share Your Passion

Just having someone that shares your fitness goals can be a huge motivation. You can work off of their energy and you can each inspire each other. When one of you are having a bad day you can rely on the other one to keep pushing you. It's like a physical trainer, but free- and better, because they're also your friend. And sometimes, simply having a friend to get active with can be enough to keep you active.

Where can you find an exercise partner?

Friend
If you have a close friend or family member who shares in your fitness goals and is about on the same fitness level as you, they can be an ideal person to make regular exercise plans with. It is important to find someone who is on a similar fitness level as you. You can keep each other motivated and can stay on par with your physical fitness growths together. Someone beneath your level is likely to hold you back, while someone above your level is likely to push your further than you can go- which can cause many people to easily get discouraged and give up. Find someone who's on the same playing field as you, and work with them to improve together.

Set a schedule with your friend or family member who'd like to exercise with you. Create a regular habit. Do not plan out spontaneously to exercise, but rather have regular meet-ups daily or weekly where you both know your schedule's will be free and you can make a point to exercise. Choose exercises you both enjoy. Sports that can be done with two people are often fantastic ways to get active often with a partner. You'll rely on the other person to show up in order to complete the exercise, which will make it a bigger priority for each of you. You'll also enjoy yourself, and if you have a competitive nature you can both push yourselves to win.

Two-Person Sports That You Can Do With Your Exercise Partner

Getting out and exercising with a partner is a great way to stay motivated. When you have someone pushing you to work harder, work longer, and get out when you don't feel like going- you are way more likely to reach your fitness goals. There are a ton of great two-person activities that you and your partner can get involved in, together.

Tennis, Racket ball: These fast paced sports only involve two people and a bit of equipment. There are free-to-access courts in many cities and towns. These sports can also be self-taught, and with a bit of practice you'll both be active in no time.

Ping-Pong: It may not seem like a super active sport, but for a slow day Ping Pong can be a fun fitness activity. Between very strenuous hard work-outs you should take a day to rest your muscles. Ping Pong can be a great get-up-and-move activity that doesn't work you both to work too hard.

Boxing/ Wrestling: Any duo fighting sport like boxing or wrestling is very physical and a great way to burn some much needed energy and stress. Be sure to take extra safety precautions so neither of you get hurt. But once you each get into the rhythm and match your skill sets, fighting activities can become a really constructive way to get physical and alleviate tension.

Exercise Ball Activities: There are a lot of activities you each can do with an exercise ball. Toss it back and forth, balancing activities, using it for strength building activities and teamwork efforts by holding it between you during workouts. Although this isn't necessarily a conventional exercise routine for two people, it's worth looking into if you want to try something new.

Volleyball: Again, this is a very active get-your-heart-pumping activity. It works out every core muscle of your body and can be done at a gym or outside. Beach volleyball is a great two person sport, because it's done on a smaller court, but still requires a ton of energy to play.

Laser Tag/ Paintball: Visit a local facility that offers one of these services and sign up as a team (or competitors!). Not only is it heart-racingly fun, it's getting you up and moving for a minimum of 30 minutes- and longer if you want your money's worth.

Even if you don't choose a two-person sport, still find an exercise activity that appeals to both of you. Take a speed-walk through the local mall, get a dual gym membership, do yoga with one another, work out at home from the comfort of your living room or get out and take a hike. Find an activity you both enjoy, find a time you both can do that activity, and schedule it in- no excuses allowed!

Spouse
Most couples, by nature, are on the same fitness level and have similar physical activity habits. Because of this your significant other can play a very healthy role in your exercise regimen. Not only do you two already know one another's schedules, chances are you live together- so it's easy to find a way to get fit with one another. It's a healthy activity that many couples can enjoy doing together. Because you've already built up a sense of honesty and support system within the relationship- transferring those same healthy habits into the way you treat one another as exercise partners. You'll be able to be truthful about fitness goals and keep each other accountable. You'll also be there

to push each other when times get tough and excuses seem easier than actions.

Make plans together, just as you would with a friend or family member, to exercise. Because you live with one another, exercising daily should be easier than it would be with any other partner. The hard part is finding the motivation to do it. If you've made a habit of not exercising with one another, getting off the couch the first few times will be difficult. But make an agreement, set a goal, and go for it. You can never get physically better together, if you never start trying to get better.

Child
Let's face it- it can be terribly hard to find a babysitter just so you can have a free moment to exercise each day. Instead of using your child for an excuse as to why you can't exercise, make them a part of your exercise regimen by making them your partner. We've already discussed an array of ways to get active with your little ones depending on their age, so let them be a part of your fitness goals. Keeping your children active and getting them involved in your physical activity is healthy and motivational for all of you.

Partner Programs
There are many partner programs available for people who want to find an exercise partner. Many local gyms have sign-ups available as well as non-profits dedicated to keeping people healthy and fit. There are also many great websites available for finding fitness partners. When searching for a partner be sure to be honest about your current fitness level, the physical activities you enjoy, and what you're hoping to get out of your time with your partner. Over-exerting yourself or falsely advertising yourself won't get you matched up with the right partner.

You want someone who's on the same level as you and has the same goals. This way, you can stay on track with one another. So be open and upfront, it will spare you both discouragement down the road.

Fitness Trainer

If you're serious about your physical activity and have the financial ability to pay a fitness trainer, having a professional who is there to keep you accountable and help you reach your fitness goals can be a great asset to you. Because they're experts in the field, they can help you get started on the right foot and make sure you're pushing your body to its limits without pushing yourself too far. They can keep you on track and help you make growth in your fitness progress.

Dog

Your canine companion might be just the push you need to get you healthy and active. Yep, that's right, beloved Toto is worth more than sloppy kisses and bedtime cuddles. Your lovable pooch can act as motivation to get you active. That little ball of fur on four legs is the best exercise friend any man could ask for.

You Have To Go Outside

Being outside, getting a breath of fresh air a couple times a day, can totally energize you and leave you feeling way more motivated to get active. When you have a dog that requires you to go outside a couple times a day to go to the bathroom, you have a forced reason to get up, get out, and self-motivate yourself multiple times. Chances are you'll come back feeling energized and ready to finish a few small active projects. You can thank Sparky's bathroom breaks for that renewed sunshine-given energy.

They Want To Walk With You
Giving your dog the best life possible requires making sure they get some exercise each day. And if they need exercise, you'll have to exercise with them. What better inspiration to get active than to have a furry creature to do it with? Taking a walk around the block twice a day will get your heart pumping and even that small feat can pay off big time in the long run. You have no excuse not to when you have a dog around. If you want the best life for your four-legged friend, you'll get up and go for a walk. Rain or shine. They deserve it and so do you.

They're Totally There, Ready To Go, When You Want To Exercise
Where else can you find an exercise companion who is ready to run any ole' time you are? Most humans aren't going to get active at your beck and call. But most dogs will. They love spending time with their human companions and are totally excited to get out and do any ole' physical activity you can come up with. They truly are your 24/7 fitness partner, just waiting around for you to say "Alright, let's go".

Ways To Stay Motivated For Your Fitness Goals

Getting fit and staying fit can be a tough feat. We all way to be in peak physical shape, but getting to and maintaining that point is difficult. We often lose sight of our goals, and lose motivation to keep going. There are ways to continue pushing through that loss of interest, if you just take the time to visualize everything. Creating a written and pictorial visual can keep you on track.

Create a picture board
Start by creating a picture board of what you want your life to look like. What does your ideal body look like- your ideal diet? Post inspiration quotes on the board, list out your reasons for wanting to get healthy. Having an imagery of where you want to be can help push you forward when you're lacking drive. If you ever feel uninspired, take a second to remember why you're doing what you're doing by looking at a collection of pictures and written pieces that define where you want to go.

Write down a yearly goal chart
Do not simply say "I'll eat healthy this month". No, plan out a year in advanced. Take a day and truly evaluate what you want to accomplish within the next year. Want to lose 100 pounds? Okay, now break that down into each month. You need to lose 9 pounds each month, that's only 2 pounds a week. Now your goal seems more manageable. How do you plan to lose 2 pounds each week? List out your goals for each week. Battle a new diet habit each month. The first month cut out soda, the second month watch your calorie intake. Focus on a different eating goal each month. Do the same thing for your exercise. Start out by wanting to run 1/2 mile a day, then the next month try running 1 mile each day. Build yourself up slowly to where you want to go.

Set reasonable goals
A big mistake that many people make is that they feel like they need to accomplish everything at once. That's not true. Success comes slowly. Set small, manageable goals that you can achieve. If you know that you can't get yourself down to 2,000 calories a day, then start at 3,500. The next month move it down to 3,000. And progressively get yourself to where you want to go.
Check off goals weekly and monthly

Every time you've achieved a goal, every time you've followed through with the plans you set yourself- mark it off on your yearly plan. Show yourself that you ARE successful and you ARE working towards your grand total. It may be a slow process, but you are making progress.

Reward yourself for goals achieved
When you do achieve a goal, reward yourself. Buy yourself a pair of jeans in a smaller size, or go out with friends and dance the night away. You are doing something awesome, and you deserve to treat yourself when you achieve what you set your mind to.

LIVING A HEALTHY LIFESTYLE FOR A LIFETIME

According to the European Journal of Social Psychology it takes 18 to 245 days to create a habit. Success in terms of living a healthy lifestyle does not come over night. It takes practice, dedication, and yes- some road blocks. It's okay to have lazy days and indulge in unhealthy treats- IN MODERATION. But being a 'fit mom' and having a healthy family starts by realizing that a majority of your lifestyle needs to be focused around healthy choices.

You CAN be 'that mom'. The one that's in shape, eats well, feeds her family well-balanced meals, and exercises regularly with her children. But, just like 'those moms' you have to make a promise to yourself and your family that that is truly a lifestyle you want to live. It can be hard work, but it doesn't have to be. Once you've made healthy living a habit, healthy living becomes something that is just a regular part of life. Make it a regular part of your life- for your kids, for your spouse, for yourself. You ARE 'The Fit Mom' starting today.

ABOUT THE AUTHOR

Dawn Walters was born April 5th 1992 and has been a foster parent since she turned twenty-one in 2013. She has currently fostered three different sibling groups totaling twelve children. She loves mothering and considers it her 'natural knack' in life. Her first book was 'A Nice Mom's Guide To Disciplining Your Child', which came after a lot of success with her online blog about her fostering adventures 'Dawn's Little Fawns' (http://dawnslittlefawns.blogspot.com). Following the publication of that book, she published her second book 'The Fit Mom'. She is currently working on her third parenting book, and is still enjoying her time as a full time foster mom.

www.ingramcontent.com/pod-product-compliance
Lightning Source LLC
Chambersburg PA
CBHW071212280526
45787CB00002B/653